T0355333

Narrative in Crisis

EXPLORATIONS IN NARRATIVE PSYCHOLOGY

MARK FREEMAN
Series Editor

BOOKS IN THE SERIES

Narrative in Crisis

Reflections from the Limits of Storytelling

Edited by

MARTIN DEGE AND IRENE STRASSER

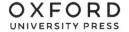

OXFORD
UNIVERSITY PRESS

Oxford University Press is a department of the University of Oxford. It furthers
the University's objective of excellence in research, scholarship, and education
by publishing worldwide. Oxford is a registered trade mark of Oxford University
Press in the UK and certain other countries.

Published in the United States of America by Oxford University Press
198 Madison Avenue, New York, NY 10016, United States of America.

Library of Congress Cataloging-in-Publication Data
Names: Dege, Martin, editor. | Strasser, Irene, 1979– editor.
Title: Narrative in crisis : reflections from the limits of storytelling /
Martin Dege & Irene Strasser.
Description: New York, NY : Oxford University Press, [2024] |
Series: Explorations in narrative psychology |
Includes bibliographical references and index.
Identifiers: LCCN 2023036656 (print) | LCCN 2023036657 (ebook) |
ISBN 9780197751756 (hardback) | ISBN 9780197751770 (epub) |
ISBN 9780197751787
Subjects: LCSH: COVID-19 Pandemic, 2020—Psychological aspects. |
Psychology—Biographical methods. | Narration (Rhetoric)—Psychological aspects.
Classification: LCC RA644.C67 N367244 2024 (print) | LCC RA644.C67 (ebook) |
DDC 616.2/4144—dc23/eng/20231018
LC record available at https://lccn.loc.gov/2023036656
LC ebook record available at https://lccn.loc.gov/2023036657

DOI: 10.1093/oso/9780197751756.001.0001

Printed by Integrated Books International, United States of America

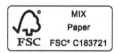

Contents

Contributors

Molly Andrews University College London, UK

Jens Brockmeier The American University of Paris, France

Martin Dege Pratt Institute, NY, USA

Michel Ferrari University of Toronto, CAN

Guro Nore Fløgstad University of South-Eastern Norway, Norway

Mark Freeman College of the Holy Cross, MA, USA

Ruthellen Josselson Fielding Graduate University, USA

Luka Lucić Pratt Institute, NY, USA

Dan P. McAdams Northwestern University, IL, USA

Hanna Meretoja University of Turku, Finland

Melanie Munroe University of Toronto, CAN

Corinne Squire School of Policy Studies, Bristol University, UK

Irene Strasser St. Bonaventure University, NY, USA

Abbreviations

AIDS	Acquired immune deficiency syndrome
AUP	American University of Paris
BKC	Bososanskim kulturnim centro (Bosnian Cultural Center)
BSE	Bovine spongiform encelphalopathy
CDC	Centers for Disease Control and Prevention (U.S.)
COVID	Coronavirus 2019
GOP	Grand Old Party (U.S. Republican Party)
HIV	Human immunodeficiency virus
IASC	Inter-Agency Standing Committee
MERS	Middle Eastern respiratory syndrome
NHS	National Health Service (UK)
PPE	Personal protective equipment
PTSD	Posttraumatic stress Disorder
SARS	Severe acute respiratory syndrome
THL	Finnish Institute for Health and Welfare
UK	United Kingdom
WHO	World Health Organization

1

Crisis Stories

Narratives of Uncertainty and Change

Irene Strasser and Martin Dege

Crises radically alter lives. The COVID-19 pandemic and its consequences on our daily lives have questioned traditional modes of practice (Castigloni & Gaj, 2020). This is true for many clinicians and practitioners but also for the academic context and the discipline of psychology. While many of us are still recovering from the collective longings to get "back to how things were before the pandemic," we have also realized that circumstances keep changing in unpredictable ways.

Crises shatter our routines and usual meaning-making in the confrontation with unexpected and uncommon events (Castigloni & Gaj, 2020). Culture usually provides baseline stories, in the background, narrating the expectable about the world and the other. If something happens outside the canonical, we are eager to make sense of it. During a crisis, "nearly everything is in violation of canonical narratives" (Josselson, Chapter 7 in this volume, p. 112). Since Spring 2020, we have become experts in administering nose swabs; we are vaccinated, boosted, and we know that the virus will not disappear anytime soon. The language has changed: from a "back to normal" expressed during large parts of the pandemic, are we now juggling the acceptance of an endemic state (Lutz & Schoenfeld Walker, 2022). Omicron (O, όμικρον), formerly innocent letter, number 15 in the Greek alphabet, will hardly recover soon from being connotated with anxiety, suffering, isolation, and, ultimately, death.

Some of the stories from the early months of the COVID-19 pandemic have moved to the background and will ultimately disappear from public discourse: that, in the beginning, experts were not sure whether mask-wearing was useful, that the sky was empty, and that air pollution decreased as international air travel significantly decreased, just as did the production of goods. Other stories we will never forget: Black Lives Matter protests during

Irene Strasser and Martin Dege, *Crisis Stories* In: *Narrative in Crisis*. Edited by: Martin Dege and Irene Strasser, Oxford University Press. © Oxford University Press 2024. DOI: 10.1093/oso/9780197751756.003.0001 the first peak of the SARS-COV-2 outbreak. People managed to show re-sistance against racism, police violence, and structural discrimination that way too many paid for with their lives. January 6, 2021, and all the political questions it brought; maybe it was images—more than stories—that shat-tered understandings of democracy and the narrative of the great and ever-progressive United States. Once more, a vast divide became visible.

In a recent study, Vanaken et al. (2021) investigated how individuals main-tain emotional well-being in times of crisis. They looked at narrative coher-ence, the extent to which narratives make sense to a listener and how they are cohesive in terms of structure and topic. Their longitudinal study started in 2018 and showed evidence that narrative coherence served as a predictor of emotional well-being during the COVID-19 pandemic. More coherent auto-biographical narratives were related to higher emotional well-being during the beginning of the pandemic (Vanaken et al., 2021). These interpretations raise essential questions. Are we successful copers if we produce *coherent* narratives? Is this genuine coping and resilience, or is it perhaps individual ignorance of uncertainty? Isn't coherency what we get from populist leaders who break down complex social dynamics into simplistic messages and easy-to-follow narratives? Isn't the clear and comprehensive slogan story of how social and behavioral measures will produce effects for everyone central to populist politics (Squire, Chapter 4 in this volume)?

We are uncertain how to structure the current crisis experiences into narratives (Andrews, Chapter 9 in this volume); not only to describe what has happened but also to describe "what is not yet but could be one day" (Meretoja, Chapter 5 in this volume, p. 83). A virus has attacked our bodies, a crisis has attacked our *selves*, while the unprecedented has attacked psy-chology (Brockmeier, Chapter 10 in this volume, p. 156), which as a disci-pline, ever since its foundation, has constantly been striving for stability. This crisis of the discipline (Dege & Strasser 2019, 2021) is moreover reflected in the general lack of public discourse contributions from psychologists to ex-plain crisis dynamics and the social implications of the COVID-19 virus and measures taken to stop its spread. As human beings and scholars, the authors of the chapters in this book ask themselves how their work matters in times of crises and how narrative research can contribute to understanding the current and ever-changing state of living, thinking, and, ultimately, coping with the "unprecedented."

Ruthellen Josselson asks what will shape the collective stories of the "end" of the pandemic once we "create a plot" (Chapter 7 in this volume, p. 122) of the COVID-19 story? Josselson reminds us that the 1920s are remembered as a time of economic prosperity and flourishing culture. The consequences of World War I and the Spanish flu were declared to have ended when the new decade—referred to as the "Roaring Twenties"—started. What are the stories we will tell—the typical narratives of the beginning 2020s? Most likely, they will be crisis narratives: the COVID-19 pandemic, Trumpism and the US Capitol attack, racist police violence, and the Russian invasion of Ukraine.

The contributions in this volume are exceptional in that they discuss crises through a theoretical and empirical lens while the authors themselves have been immersed in ongoing states of crisis: the current COVID-19 pandemic and the scholarly, academic crisis of psychology. Thus, with this volume, we aim to contribute to discussions that only have begun as part of rethinking psychologies. The chapters of this volume discuss different aspects of crisis dynamics: *narratives of inequality*, narratives as ways to approach *the unprecedented*, narratives of navigating *uncertainty*, and narratives about *us and the other*.

Narratives of Inequality

The current crises illuminate once more social inequality as well as increased disparities and bring to the fore new forms of inequality (Bambra et al., 2020; Marmot & Allen, 2020; Strasser & Dege, 2021). Early in 2020, while several leaders of the political West still struggled to acknowledge the pandemic state of the COVID-19 crisis, many intellectuals had already started voicing their concerns that "America was facing a racial pandemic within the viral pandemic" (Kendi, 2020). Nevertheless, different "lifestyles" and health behavior were blamed for the fact that members of racialized ethnic minorities, specifically African American citizens, were more likely to be infected with COVID-19, were more likely to suffer severe outcomes and death. COVID-19 forced us to recognize—once again—the conditions of racialized necropolitics and health inequalities that produce so-called pre-existing health conditions and systematically put members of marginalized groups at a disadvantage (Sandset, 2021). Long before the crises of this decade, Butler (2016), Mbembe (2019), and others started to discuss the need to look into the politics of whose lives seem to count and are grievable as we are confronted with the significant impact of racial politics and their "necropolitical underpinnings" (Sandset, 2021). Not only do we not hear certain voices, but we also do not see certain bodies—we face an abjection of non-normative bodies during times of the pandemic (Núñez-Parra et al., 2021, p. 544).

"We are all in this together" emerged as a possible master narratives of the pandemic at an early stage of realizing the global impact of COVID-19. Unlike Ebola, Zika, and the swine flu, this time the so-called Global North faced a pandemic, a severe health threat caused by a virus much harder to control than human immunodeficiency virus (HIV) several decades ago. Only, "we" were never really in this together. From the very beginning, there were incremental differences in available resources and agency that determined how well individuals were capable of dealing with situations like lockdowns, quarantines, and health preventive requirements. It became a consumerist endeavor to protect oneself by staying safe—purchasing protective gear, having health insurance to get tested, and, ultimately, having the ability to work remotely in one's home rather than in a shared office or production facility. The fact that everyone was a potential patient in this pandemic (Meretoja, Chapter 5 in this volume) still produced very different risks and outcomes for different groups of individuals in different corners of the world. "Narratives are entangled with power," Meretoja reminds us (p. 71), and it is a matter of positionality and intersectionality that determines whose COVID narratives are acknowledged and included in public discourse and empirical research. Untold stories of loss (Josselson, Chapter 7 in this volume) join the chorus of unheard stories. And while many could afford to have hope of soon getting "back to normal," some started to voice concerns "that normal wasn't so great for lots of people" (Freeman, Chapter 2 in this volume, p. 31) and doubted a soon-to-be post-pandemic world (Squire, Chapter 4 in this volume).

Will we have learned something about humanity and equality after this pandemic has ended? Who pronounces such an end, and to what ends? Did we ever believe that the virus—a biological entity first described in late 2019—would finally disappear, together with the devastating effects of pandemic and austerity politics, including further disparity in the health system (Strasser & Dege, 2021)?

Unprecedented Times

The disruptions caused by the pandemic—more so, the human-made consequences of the measures taken or not taken—have significantly impacted individuals and communities. Individuals cope differently with crises (Todorova et al., 2021). "Some people stop watching the news. Some turn to other things," Freeman states (Chapter 2 in this volume, p. 25). However, many deal with changes and challenges because there seems to be no alternative. From a traditional psychological perspective, the emphasis would be on individualized resilience and the ideal of personal growth through difficult life experiences. But we need to ask critically: Do we really grow from crisis experiences like the COVID-19 pandemic? Do we experience growth in the sense that it helps individuals and communities to be better prepared for future crises?

McAdams reminds us of Ancient Greek and Shakespearian theater, where "the hero learns that suffering is unavoidable in life" (Chapter 3 in this volume, p. 47) and refers to Camus's *Plague*: Dr. Rieux, as narrator, "wants us to know that the very same human story might apply across the board in many different times and places" (p. 46). After all, we might come to the conclusion that crises like the COVID-19 pandemic are not so much unprecedented as unpredictable. Understanding history as "a record of human intentionality" (Josselson, Chapter 7 in this volume, p. 122), it is the stories of uncertain times and helplessness that become untold stories or, as Josselson remarks in reference to Bollas, "unthought knowns." As such, the notion of the *unprecedented* retakes center stage, even though we have lived through moments of crisis before. Meretoja points us to the application of specific language in moments of global crisis: we use war metaphors to find words for something that is not-so-unprecedented (Chapter 5 in this volume). What started to be publicly referred to as the three Cs—*conflict, climate,* and *COVID-19*— constitute the beginning of the 2020s, with the list of conflicts expanding: the Russian war against Ukraine, a conservative battle against women's rights in the United States, backlash climate politics and an energy crisis in Europe, starvation in sub-Saharan Africa.

The development of vaccines, their side effects, and related statistics have been discussed extensively in public discourse. At the same time, we got an insight into epistemological practices in science, into the "randomized controlled trials" on the one hand and the "trial-and-error style" of building knowledge on the other. And, rather than idealizing biomedical and psychological research as if it was an exact science, many started to realize that those analyses "are always provisional" (Andrews, Chapter 9 in this volume, p. 140).

But what do we learn, and how do we grow from what happens, both individually and collectively (Ferrari & Munroe, Chapter 8 in this volume)?

When not being able to deal with the unknown we, as individuals, tend to seek reassurance in the thought that we might go back to something that we know (Josselson, Chapter 7 in this volume). Several (former) political leaders like Trump, Johnson, Bolsonaro, Putin, etc. refused to acknowledge an uncertain reality; instead, they subscribed to magical thinking as a strategy to deal with the out-of-control situation (Andrews, Chapter 9 in this volume). This is a typical right-wing populist strategy that resonates with many in their audiences, as people seem tempted by the "lure of narrative" (Freeman, Chapter 2 in this volume). And, over time, we got used to this infantilization through simplistic messages about the virus and related measures.

"Mask up!," "No mask, no service!," "Make sure your mask fits properly!," "Mask up and carry on!," "Need a mask? Just ask!" Hardly ever do we hear about the fact that we primarily wear masks to protect "the other"'—not ourselves. And that the Trump supporters' anti-mask parole "my body, my choice"'—referring to masks, not abortion rights—jeopardized others' health, not their own. Trump himself, over the course of his pandemic presidency, was, as McAdams puts it, "psychologically unable to articulate a long-term plan to address the pandemic" (Chapter 3 in this volume, p. 39). For some people, listening to *narratives of messianic fashion* (Freeman, Chapter 2 in this volume) seems to have become the turn-to coping strategy contra uncertainty.

Narratives of Uncertainty and Change

As scholars, many of us did not know how to explain what was going on, specifically at the beginning of the pandemic and with the lack of appropriate data. Josselson impressively points out her struggle with not having data and, therefore, not-knowing (Chapter 7 in this volume). Many questioned the extent to which we do *not* know the virus and how lives will continue, and they started to question things we had taken for granted (Andrews, in this volume). While we continue to gain more insight in hindsight (Freeman, 2010), we also continue to stumble over what the future holds for us: new variants, new vaccines, new ways of social interactions, new mandates, new unprecedented restrictions and other measures, or, eventually, the radical acceptance (McAdams, Chapter 3 in this volume) that this state of uncertainty will not go away any time soon. The more widespread way of dealing with uncertainty seems to be to reduce heterogeneity into singularity, that is, to point the finger at the unwelcome "other" as responsible for the crisis (Freeman, Chapter 2 in this volume)—the refugee, the intellectual, the virus. In crises, particularly, it seems appealing to reach for a story that helps reduce ambivalence and pretends certainty.

Greenhalgh et al. (2021) show how, early in the pandemic, scientists publicly discussed the droplet mode of transmission versus the airborne mode of transmission. Either way, the narratives always tried to imply certainty about what is scientifically correct. The authors argue that pandemic policymaking involves "competing narratives" (p. 1)—essentially, a competition between science and moral narratives—in an attempt to disguise scientific uncertainty. In the face of an ambiguous, limited, and uncertain world (McAdams, Chapter 3 in this volume), our lives seem "governed by an illusion of control" (Meretoja, Chapter 5 in this volume, p. 76).

During the pandemic, we used the term "crises" for different yet related events: the COVID-related aspects of the pandemic; the protests following the murder of George Floyd and the relationship between colonialism, systemic racism, and police violence (Bamberg, 2021); the war in Ukraine; the disrupted supplies of energy and food. Instead of discussing "crisis," Bamberg suggests "uncertainty" as a more useful concept to uncover the fact that we are not merely facing a temporary instability but rather a novel state—one "that has no clear beginning nor ending" (Bamberg, 2021, p. 62). Eventually, in early 2022, when mask and vaccine mandates were dropped amid the highest numbers of infection ever, many finally had come to terms with the idea that "the virus never fully goes away [...] but must be managed" (McAdams, Chapter 3 in this volume, p. 36).

The Other

Beyond the aforementioned simplistic parole of "us all being in this together," this pandemic repeatedly produced discourses of "othering." Indeed, the other as a potential threat seems to be one of the dominant narratives. While it was true for potentially everyone that they might become a threat to another person by having contracted the virus and pass it on, some groups were not even acknowledged as subjects who may become threats but instead were entirely stripped of their agency. This is exemplified in narratives of the vulnerable older adult, whom we supposedly have to protect from themselves. After realizing that vaccines do not completely stop the spread but do decrease the individual risk of severe illness, some countries discussed or even passed laws that require citizens above a certain age to get vaccinated (Amante et al., 2022; German lawmakers reject vaccine, 2022).

Beyond normative dimensions of development, psychologists investigate autobiographical narratives to understand how we have become who we are and what makes one more likely to frame redemptive stories (McAdams, 2012), that is, stories that transform negative events into more positive endings. We could keep our hopes up that this pandemic, with all its negative consequences on the individual and societal levels, will produce such redemptive narratives that eventually unfold the potential to make the world a better place, where we use narrative imagination to learn from the crisis (Andrews, Chapter 9 and Meretoja, Chapter 5 in this volume). At the same time, the COVID crisis produced narratives using war metaphors in manifold ways. Stories about the virus as an entity that "attacks" us and "frontline workers" (medical staff) who "fight back" long dominated the pandemic discourse. However, those stories are not necessarily supportive nor appreciative of the difficult work that individuals performed in the health sector, with many of them having paid with their lives (Meretoja, Chapter 5 in this volume): "The narrative of war heroism justifies putting health workers at risk" (p. 74), and political leaders benefit from it.

On a more general level, we might ask what kind of perspective, what kind of coping and collective resilience we need as a society to produce redemptive stories. Will shared experiences of feeling disconnected (isolation, lockdowns, quarantines) create an understanding of "shared interconnectedness" (Freeman, Chapter 2 in this volume, p. 16)? And even if that was the case for the immediate time of lockdowns and other pandemic measures, how would we preserve the stories and feelings of connectedness?

Crisis Narratives

The *virus* attacks the body, *crisis* attacks the self and thereby brings it to the fore, and the *unprecedented* attacks psychology (Brockmeier, Chapter 10 in this volume) because it is founded on ideals of constancy and stability—despite its desire for growth and change (Dege & Strasser, 2019).

In this volume, distinguished scholars of narrative provide their early attempts—triggered by the COVID-19 pandemic—to understand "crises" from a narrative perspective. They discuss the narrative notions of crises as an ongoing situation, thereby uncovering ideals of stability and certainty as epistemologically questionable psychological concepts. The authors all start with insight into early considerations, from mid-2020, at a time still without vaccines and variants. They revisit their thoughts over the course of the ongoing pandemic and relate their research perspective to autoethnographic and biographical approaches to "crisis narratives." As scholars and citizens, they share vulnerable moments of uncertainty—what we don't know and will not know—and they draw on past collective experiences. What did we learn from the Spanish flu? How well do experts and journalists really understand what those numbers are supposed to signify? How unparalleled is the unprecedented experience for individuals who have experienced war, sieges (Lucić & Fløgstad, Chapter 6 in this volume), and previous pandemics? And, finally, will we ever learn to live with the virus?

The chapters shed light on ambiguities relating to us and the other, rational and irrational approaches to navigating crises, and other ambivalences without aiming to solve them. They investigate levels of the individual, academic work, and society and highlight stories of the unknown or yet-to-be known (Josselson, Chapter 7 and Meretoja, Chapter 5 in this volume) by making them accessible through thorough reflection, pushing back the all-too-simplified stories we hear in everyday discourses.

Part I of the volume questions the power of narrative. For a long time in the development of narrative psychology, researchers emphasized the potential of a narrative viewpoint. Beyond the analysis of life stories, the narrative perspective developed a better grasp of everyday meaning-making processes, identity formation, political movements, and a plethora of other aspects. The COVID-19 crisis and its politics, including the application of "narrative" to bend facts and invent truths, force narrative researchers to question their stance on narrative as a largely liberating and enabling concept. The authors in this section explore narrative from this critical point of view and deliberate the limits of the narrative perspective or pitfalls that might have been overlooked in the past. Mark Freeman (Chapter 2 of this book) emphasizes the "lure" of narrative and discusses the relationship between information, misinformation, and disinformation in times of crisis. Dan McAdams (Chapter 3) uses Camus's *Plague* to discuss different narratives of making sense of the COVID-19 pandemic. Corinne Squire (Chapter 4) looks at dominant political narratives and policy discourses as well as counteracting narratives and how they potentially create moments of solidarity. Hanna Meretoja (Chapter 5) discusses how COVID-19 public images are framed with war narratives that provide us with illusions of agency and control. Luka Lucić and Guro Nore Fløgstad (Chapter 6) research narratives of young people who grew up during the siege of Sarajevo in the 1990s and point out complex psychological responses beyond individual trauma narratives.

The contributions in Part II of this volume discuss self and identity in the middle of uncertain times. How do individuals experience a sudden loss of perspective for their future? What is the effect of losing control over various aspects of everyday life? How is the self affected by such abrupt and unexpected changes that result in a largely unforeseeable future? Beyond reflections on a loss of stability, the chapters in this part of the volume dare to explore potential lessons we might learn from this pandemic and ask how this will allow us to be better equipped for future uncertainties. Ruthellen Josselson (Chapter 7) discusses the disintegration of life due to crisis and asks what we know and what we can know in the face of the pandemic. Michel Ferrari and Melanie Munroe (Chapter 8) look at coping strategies during crises and specifically examine whether a crisis constitutes a decisive state or a turning point. Molly Andrews (Chapter 9) examines how we are reimagining our lives during the COVID-19 crisis and frames the pandemic as a failure of the narrative imagination. Finally, Jens Brockmeier (Chapter 10) investigates the omnipresence of the self in crises narratives and the potential crisis of the self implied therein; a crisis that draws from the struggle for meaning that we need to take beyond a war against an outside threat.

References

Amante, A., Fonte, G., & Jones, G. (2022, January 6). Italy extends COVID vaccine mandate to everyone over 50. *Reuters*. https://www.reuters.com/world/europe/italy-make-covid-jab-mandatory-over-50s-tighten-curbs-draft-2022-01-05/

Bamberg, M. (2021). Uncertainty—What Pfizer, Billy Graham, Trump, and psychology have in common. In M. Dege & I. Strasser (Eds.), *Global Pandemics and Epistemic Crises in Psychology: A Socio-Philosophical Approach* (pp. 59–71).

Bambra, C., Riordan, R., Ford, J., & Matthews, F. (2020). The COVID-19 pandemic and health inequalities. *Journal of Epidemiology and Community Health, jech-2020*. https://doi.org/10.1136/jech-2020-214401

Butler, J. (2016). *Frames of war: When is life grievable?* Verso.

Castiglioni, M., & Gaj, N. (2020). Fostering the reconstruction of meaning among the general population during the covid-19 pandemic. *Frontiers in Psychology, 11*. https://doi.org/10.3389/fpsyg.2020.567419

Dege, M., & Strasser, I. (2019). The Lone Wolf Coder: An autoethnographic reflection on the International Congress of Qualitative Inquiry in Urbana-Champaign, Illinois. *Human Arenas, 2*(3), 322–340.

Dege, M., & Strasser, I. (Eds.). (2021). *Global pandemics and epistemic crises in psychology: A socio-philosophical approach*. Routledge

Freeman, M. (2010). *Hindsight: The promise and peril of looking backward*. Oxford University Press.

German lawmakers reject vaccine mandate for people over 60. (2022, April 7). *DW*. https://www.dw.com/en/german-lawmakers-reject-vaccine-mandate-for-people-over-60/a-61387119

Greenhalgh, T., Ozbilgin, M., & Tomlinson, D. (2021). How COVID-19 spreads: Narratives, counter-narratives, and social dramas. Authorea. November 2021. https://doi.org/10.22541/au.163709155.56570215/v1

Kendi, I. X. (2020, April 14). Stop blaming black people for dying of the coronavirus: New data from 29 states confirm the extent of the racial disparities. *The Atlantic*. https://www.theatlantic.com/ideas/archive/2020/04/race-and-blame/609946/

Lutz, E., & Schoenfeld Walker, A. (2022, April 7). Is this what endemic disease looks like? *The New York Times*. https://www.nytimes.com/interactive/2022/04/07/science/endemic-meaning-pandemic-covid.html

Marmot, M., & Allen, J. J. (2020). COVID-19: Exposing and amplifying inequalities. *Journal of Epidemiology and Community Health, 74*, 681–682

McAdams, D. P. (2012). Exploring psychological themes through life-narrative accounts. In J. A. Holstein & J. F. Gubrium (Eds.), *Varieties of Narrative Analysis* (pp. 15–32). Sage.

Mbembe, A. (2019). *Necropolitics*. Duke University Press.

Núñez-Parra, L., López-Radrigán, C., Mazzucchelli, N., & Pérez C. (2021). Necropolitics and the bodies that do not matter in pandemic times. *Alter – European Journal of Disability Research/Revue Européenne de Recherche Sur le Handicap, 15*, 190–197.

Sandset, T. (2021). The necropolitics of COVID-19: Race, class and slow death in an ongoing pandemic. *Global Public Health, 16*(8–9), 1411–1423. https://doi.org/10.1080/17441692.2021.1906927

Strasser, I., & Dege, M. (2021). Crises, politics, psychology: An introduction. In I. Strasser & M. Dege (Eds.), *The psychology of global crises and crisis politics: Intervention, resistance, decolonization* (pp. 1–18). Palgrave.

Todorova, I., Albers, L., Aronson, N., Baban, A., Benyamini, Y., Cipolletta, S., Del Rio Carral, M., Dimitrova, E., Dudley, C., Guzzardo, M., Hammoud, R., Fadil Azim, D. H., Hilverda, F., Huang, Q., John, L., Kaneva, M., Khan, S., Kostova, Z., Kotzeva, T., . . . Patel, H. (2021). "What I thought was so important isn't really that important": International perspectives on making meaning during the first wave of the COVID-19 pandemic. *Health Psychology and Behavioral Medicine, 9*(1), 830–857. https://doi.org/10.1080/21642850.2021.1981909

Vanaken, L., Bijttebier, P., Fivush, R., & Hermans, D. (2021). Narrative coherence predicts emotional well-being during the COVID-19 pandemic: A two-year longitudinal study. *Cognition and Emotion, 36*(1), 70–81. https://doi.org/10.1080/02699931.2021.1902283

PART I
END OF STORY?

2

The (Al)lure of Narrative

Information, Misinformation, and Disinformation in the Time of Coronavirus

Mark Freeman

Hope, Despair, Nausea

My task in this chapter is a difficult one, mainly because a good chunk of time has passed since the Psychology of Global Crises conference, at which I presented an initial version of these ideas. That was May 2020. Covid was still in dreadfully high gear, George Floyd had just been murdered, and Donald Trump was continuing his reign of idiocy, hopeful that he would sail through the election and debase the United States for another four years. Through it all, many at the conference insisted on adopting a stance of hopefulness, even optimism, their hope (wish?) being that people's encounter with pandemic life—or at least the life of those who weren't actually the victims of the pandemic—would lead to some salutary existential reorientations. They, we, would pause and take stock, perhaps think anew about some of our pre-pandemic commitments, shift our priorities. We would gather a clear sense of life's preciousness and become more cognizant of the incredible care and love that were being displayed among healthcare workers and the like. We would see how vital their contributions were, and have always been, to our collective well-being, and we would let them know, too. I was attracted to these possibilities, too. But, if truth be told, I was in a darker, more fearful place. I will try to convey some of this in the pages that follow if only to high-light some of the dynamics of the time. But, of course, now that I know what has gone on since that fateful time—including, among other things, the presidential campaign, Donald Trump's loss, the siege on the Capitol steps, and the sheer lunacy that has followed in its wake, especially among those previously thought to have above-average intelligence—I find myself in still darker place now. Once it was clear (to sane people) that Donald Trump had

Mark Freeman, *The (Al)lure of Narrative* In: *Narrative in Crisis*. Edited by: Martin Dege and Irene Strasser, Oxford University Press. © Oxford University Press 2024. DOI: 10.1093/oso/9780197751756.003.0002 lost the election, and, once people bore witness to the savagery on the Capitol steps, one might have assumed that the awful chapter in question was over, or at least in retreat. I guess that was my hope (wish?). Silly me.

But let me return to the conference and the hope that pervaded much of it. A number of speakers at the conference suggested, rightly, that catastrophic events of the sort we were seeing at the time could yield new forms of care and solidarity, even *communitas* (Turner, 1995), a coming-together in the face of liminality, an intimate sharing of a sort that might not have been possible without the catastrophe at hand. Something like this emerged in the wake of 9/11 in the States; in Banda Aceh, Indonesia, following the tsunami that hit some years back; and following many other such events. In some of my own work, I have acknowledged this phenomenon under the rubric of "the priority of the Other" (Freeman, 2014), especially the person in need who calls forth my care. It's possible, I wrote at the time, that this "centrifugal" sense of caring and relational solidarity, this being-called-outward, beyond the self, beyond the ego, will be long-lasting; it's possible that something was *revealed* about our shared humanity, our shared interconnectedness, and that it will have staying power. *Eros*, Freud (1930/1962]) called it, the power of love, the power of binding people together into larger wholes—families, communities, even nations. This sort of "wake-up" call can happen on the personal plane, too: in the face of a debilitating, dangerous disease, one may confront and even embrace one's own vulnerability and mortality and live differently. It's also possible, I ventured, that these sorts of revelations will lead us to theorize in new, more appropriately relational ways.

I shared these forms of hope with many of the people at this conference, and I, like them, saw that moment as a real opportunity to think and live differently, beyond the sovereign, seemingly self-sufficient self. I did, however, voice some worries about its staying power. That's because there is often a kind of "reversion" backward after the initial rush, a centripetal return to what I (Freeman, 2014) have referred to as the "ordinary oblivion," the forgetfulness, of everyday life. In this respect, I had said, I think we have both an opportunity and a challenge: the challenge of *remembering*, of keeping in view these different ways of thinking and living and being.

I also worried about the fact that the kind of solidarity some had spoken of isn't the only form of it. As has become all too clear—in the wake of Capitol siege, most visibly, but also in the form of the dogged, stubborn, evidence-free claims of anti-vaxxers, who, remarkably, seem intent on bringing about their own untimely deaths—there are quite negative forms, too, ones that are sometimes pitted against the positive ones, culminating in ugly modes of Us/ Them thinking.

This brings me to a related thought, which I want to offer cautiously. During the course of listening to some of the more hopeful, forward-looking talks that were presented at the conference, it dawned on me that none of them was from the United States, where both the medical—and especially the political—situation had been, and remains, truly horrifying. There are, of course, people who have a hopeful vision here, too, but it's mainly among those who can afford to hope, so to speak, who have the "luxury" of hope. I don't mean this as a criticism of the vision. But I do think the nature and magnitude of hope are distributed unevenly, at least in the States, in line with extant class differences, inequalities, and so on. This isn't a reason not to hope; there is always a reason to hope (as long as we distinguish it from optimism, which remains in short supply). But it is a reason to continue to recognize the hopeless and despairing. There are many.

Where did these preliminary comments lead me? Well, they led me to a somewhat more suspicious and fearful image of the future and to a kind of vigilance regarding what was happening at the time and what might happen going forward. Alongside *Eros*, Freud (1930/1962) told us, is *Thanatos*, the power of death, of undoing and perhaps destroying what binds us together. This was a curious place for me to be. I usually land on the brighter, more upbeat side of things. In better moments, I still land there. But at that particular moment, I found myself wanting to supplement the more positive visions that had been offered with a kind of counterweight, one that would return us to the gravity and urgency of the current situation. The last thing I would want to do here, now, is gloat or claim some sort of prophecy. Hardly; as far as I could tell, the writing was on the wall. And what it essentially said is: Beware. We are in some deep shit. As indeed we were. And are. And, at the heart of it all, on some level, is narrative.

This may seem like a too-large claim. Given what was going on at the time and given what is still going on in the States, there are other heart-of-it-all contenders: tribalism, gullibility, resentment, mistrust, and, not least, ignorance and stupidity. All of these are, arguably, "prior" to narrative. But they wouldn't, and couldn't, have taken hold in the way they have without narrative. Our man Donald Trump wants us to guzzle disinfectant? Will do! We can take a drug intended for livestock (Ivermectin) and root out little COVID critters? Why not? But maybe there is no need to even go this far. It could be that it's all a hoax! Same for the election of Joe Biden. The Big Lie! Well, some might say in response to all this snarkiness, there's always going to be a group of people who fall prey to these kinds of storylines. But Reason will surely win out. Well, not quite. In January 2022, still many hospitals are filled to capacity with the unvaccinated. Who are all you left-wing socialists to tell *me* what I am required to inject into my body? My body my self! Except, of course, if we're talking about abortion. These people are taking the beds of those in urgent need of medical care, and some of them are dying as a result. As for the election, approximately two-thirds of Republican voters still believe it was stolen. From their hero—a despicable human being if there ever was one. Much of this is flat-out mystifying, at least for "my kind." It's maddening as well.

How Did We Get Here?

In what follows, I chart three somewhat distinct phases of my own thinking about these issues, phases that basically parallel what has been going on in the States since Donald Trump entered the picture. I don't want to talk about him much, mainly because I don't want to give him undue attention; he has taken enough from us already, and I don't want to give him much more. In any case, on to the phases.

I will call Phase One the *serious concerns* phase. The first piece I did on these issues took the form of a lecture I gave at the American University of Paris, at the kind invitation of Brian Schiff. Titled "Whose story? Whose world? Life and narrative in the age of Trump," I gave that talk about a month after Trump's inauguration—the one where he fantasized, or hallucinated, or simply *lied*, about the massive crowd that had gathered to hear his incredible words. Here is a passage from the talk (Freeman, 2017).

We're experiencing what might be called *narrative anxiety*. A story is unfolding, that much is clear, but we don't know yet what it is. And that's very, very scary. Sometimes this story-in-the-making seems to be one of a brash and bumbling narcissistic incompetent who's getting so frustrated by the relentless criticisms he himself is bringing upon himself that he's bound to implode and maybe just give up or do something so outlandish that he'll be impeached. Unfortunately, this seems unlikely to me, mainly because of his clear and obvious loathing of failure, coupled with his truly remarkable powers of fictional transformation. Somehow, he was able to turn paltry crowds the day of inauguration into teeming masses, clamoring, joyfully, for their new leader. Now, rationally speaking, one might assume that he knew, in his heart, that it wasn't such a great showing and just did a little psychological maneuvering in order to reassure himself and his followers that the event was a rousing success. This would be a fairly standard psychodynamic narrative: a little denial, a little wishful thinking, and *voila*, a huge crowd. And maybe when he sat on the edge of his king-size bed that night, ready to crawl in with Melania, he had a moment of painful self-confrontation. "Geez, that was kind of pathetic." More likely, though—that is, if he could admit that the turnout was a whole lot sparser than he'd wished—he'd be enraged and point to all the evil people, in the media especially, who drove away the crowds and thereby prevented him from gaining the glory that was rightfully his. This would be a standard narrative, too: frustrated with his poor, utterly unfair treatment, the victim rails against those hell-bent on destroying him. This one's a bit more plausible, mainly because of the narcissistic-assault-and-rage angle. "I *hate* them all!" he might have said. "I want them *out*! And then, a solution. "Let me get rid of who I can . . . "

It wasn't long after I shared these words that Trump began addressing the so-called border crisis, the extrusion of the unwelcome Other serving as a particularly alluring storyline for those wishing to make America great again: pure, unsullied, *white*. It also wasn't too long after that that there would be further exclusions and extrusions, essentially of anyone who threatened the narrative-in-the-making by either criticizing him or speaking the truth. We might think of this as *narrative cleansing*—or, maybe better still, *narrative whitewashing*—such that all the ugly stories of his incompetence and corruptness, along with all the people who told them, would be purged. This went on throughout Trump's entire term as President and resulted in the dismissal of a number of people who dared to speak the truth.

As an aside, it's interesting that many of those sympathetic to constructionist or even poststructuralist thinking suddenly found themselves being realists, calling out lies for what they were, refusing interpretive relativism and inane conspiracy theories. "Not true!" many of "our kind," said. "People died in the Capitol siege. You can't construct reality however you want!" It's also interesting, of course, that those on the proverbial other side (for now, I'm assuming most of the people who read this sort of chapter are fellow travelers), who often decried interpretive relativism and pushed their own reified forms of scientific thinking, ought to have become would-be constructionists. "You think the Capitol siege was a violent insurrection," some have said. "I see it as an FBI hoax" (or a peaceful patriotic protest or a day of touristic sightseeing, etc.). A strange turnabout, this one.

But let me return to the larger issues. So far, I have been discussing Trump and some of the things he did and continues to do to sustain his image and storyline. But we shouldn't forget that it takes *audiences*, "readers," to keep storylines alive. What is, again, so strange and mystifying, at least to lots of the people I tend to hang with, is that the more Trump's absurdities and lies and outright horrors emerged, the more solidified his base became. Apparently, there was no room for complexity or multiplicity. Many people didn't seem to care about Trump-the-racist or Trump-the-misogynist or the many sordid tales that emerged throughout his term and afterward. And, even if they did care, they seem to have found it perilously easy to sweep it all aside and do some cleansing and purging of their own. These were people who were so disgusted with politics as usual or so contemptuous of some of the players involved that they seem to have been willing to give Trump a pass in the hope that this utterly different kind of character could bring some much-needed change to politics and to their lives. There were also those whose support was born out of pure self-interest, whether political or economic or both. These were the "hold your nose" people, people who knew full well what was going on but felt they had to stay the course, whether in the hope that their meager coffers might get filled or their already-stuffed ones might get fuller.

Other people, it should be noted, identified with Trump: the intrepid iconoclast who tells it like it is, who's there, for *us*, to undo all the niceties of politics-as-usual. That's still the case. Others felt disenfranchised or ignored. That, at least, was one of the leading narratives in the aftermath of the election. "He's still our guy," some of them said. In addition, as a friend of mine who read an initial draft of this chapter reminded me, there were the "one-issue" people, the people so committed to one issue—abortion, gun control, immigration, Israel, whatever—that everything else was incidental, a mere blip on the screen of their unswerving single-mindedness. All of this is by way of saying that was a lot going on besides the allure of narrative, and it's important to acknowledge it.

But the allure was real. In that initial talk I gave, I went on to identify three distinct narrative dangers. The first, which fits scarily well with the one-issue idea, is what I called *narrative homogenization*, the reduction of multiplicity into singularity. We saw this in full bloom in the crisis over the border wall, which, on Trump's account, portrayed the immigrant border-crosser as a dangerous intruder, lurking on our doorsteps, or as a useless, skill-less parasite or thief, stealing from the natives. Lock the doors. Put up fences. Build walls. These two storylines—and there are others—are variations on the theme I spoke of earlier: the extrusion of the unwelcome Other, so as to preserve the purity and the primacy of the Same.

We saw a variant of these storylines in how Trump and his minions handled the more recent unwelcome Other, the coronavirus crisis. It's no big deal, Trump essentially said at the beginning. On January 22, 2020, there was one confirmed case in the States. "We do have a plan," he said, "and we think it's gonna be handled very well, we've already handled it very well." No worries. Shortly after, a second case was confirmed. A week later, there were five cases. Eventually, the World Health Organization declared coronavirus a public health emergency. But to all the alarmists still out there: *Relax.* "We think we have it very well under control," Trump said the next day. "We have very little problem in this country at this moment—five—and those people are all recuperating successfully." So, "we think it's going to have a very good ending for us . . . that I can assure you." The protector, the reassurer. Leaping ahead to February 26, Trump said, "You have 15 people, and the 15 within a couple of days is going to be down to close to zero." This might be called the "Whew!" or "Close call!" narrative. Thank goodness *that's* out of the way. . . .

Eventually, Trump would actually say, "We have met the moment and we have prevailed." That was on the day the death toll in the States passed 80,000. "We will transition into greatness," he would eventually add. "That's a phrase you're going to hear a lot." He was right about that. *Narrative homogenization*, revisited, even in the face of indisputable facts pointing in the direction of other, more truthful narratives entirely. As many experts said at the time, the facts suggest that the administration's response to the coronavirus was an utter disaster and involved insufficient testing, failure to send needed medical gear to healthcare workers, cutting off funding to the World Health Organization, firing experts who sought to speak the truth, and spreading bizarre misinformation along with some flat-out lies, most of which either blamed others for what went on or called for gratitude and appreciation in light of the great good that had been done. "It's profoundly painful," I said in the conference talk (Freeman, 2020).

> Every single day. It's also monumentally absurd—at least to those of us who think it's monumentally absurd. And again, what's astounding and mystifying, is that Trump and his obsequious imprinting-style ducklings

can do all of this and his approval rating continues to approach 50%. I want to try to understand it.

In February 2022, the death toll in the United States is more than ten times what it was at the time. And the lion's share of the newly dead come from the legions of the unvaccinated. Some anti-vaxxers or vaccine skeptics have justifiable reasons for their wariness or refusal: African Americans, for instance, may be all too aware of the ways in which their ancestors were abused in the name of research. But for many, the reasons are much more ideological. The "imprinting-style ducklings" metaphor isn't quite right in this context. Lemmings is more like it. As the New Hampshire motto has it, "Live free or die." How tragic that "freedom" ought to have been reduced to this. And how deadly.

I don't want to get too self-righteous framing things in the way I have. Nor do I want to just move into contempt mode, tempting though that is. A quick story in this context: every now and then, I rail against someone who does something asinine—in traffic, for instance, or at the grocery store—and say something like, "Must be a Trumper." Or must be a friend of Mitch McConnell. Whatever. One of our daughters, who knows and quite likes some card-carrying Trumpers, is quick to offer a kind of rebuke of such crude, stereotyped images of who these people are. "Most of the people I know are good people," she might say. "They just have different views about things than you do." So chill out, you arrogant lefty, she's essentially saying, and have some respect for people who are different from you. I actually think that what she has to say in this context is admirable. It's certainly more charitable. While I am ready to either explode in rage or implode in despair, she, with her live-and-let-live stance, continues to welcome the stranger, so to speak, into her midst. She is no fan of Trump, mind you, and she's gotten her vaccinations, booster, and so on. She just won't go into high critical/contempt mode with his supporters, at least not in the blanket way I and others sometimes do. Good for her. My blood pressure went up this year; I have a trusty measuring device sitting nearby. Hers is probably fine.

But I still want to know: How is it possible? It's not just a matter of different views. For some, it appears to be a flagrant denial of reality or, less severely (but no less problematically), a flagrant *disregard* for it, a condition of being so ensconced in an ideological position as to effectively say, "I don't *care* about reality. I'm willing to go with the narrative no matter what." Molly Andrews, in her conference talk, also mentioned *resistance* to reality, resistance to *knowing*—"willed ignorance," as Primo Levi (1989) has called it. As noted earlier, there is also the fetishization of individualism and freedom. So, I don't want to oversimplify things. But I still want to know: How is it possible? How is it possible for misinformation and disinformation to nullify real information grounded in some semblance of reality?

Alongside the idea of narrative homogenization, I had also put forth the related idea of *narrative apocalypticism*, which referred to the kind of totalizing narrative that entailed the destruction of the established order and its replacement by a new one, a *greater* one, one that promised an unprecedented opportunity for redemption and salvation. Some may recall some of the now infamous words uttered at Trump's (2017) inauguration speech when he referred to

> mothers and children trapped in poverty in our inner cities; rusted out factories scattered like tombstones across the landscape of our nation; an education system flush with cash, but which leaves our young and beautiful students deprived of all knowledge; and the crime and the gangs and the drugs that have stolen too many lives and robbed our country of so much unrealized potential.

"This American carnage stops right here and stops right now," he went on to say, and he, of course, was the One to make it happen. As for what was going on beyond our own borders, we were also going to take on "radical Islamic terrorism, which we will eradicate from the face of the Earth" (Trump, 2017).

Along these lines, there is no question but that, for many, Trump's appeal is a religious one, tied to purification and salvation. Trump knew how to tell this story, and, in true messianic fashion, he gathered a big and devoted flock along the way—including, but by no means limited to, those evangelicals who, out of their deep religious fervor, were willing to follow his lead. That flock is still there. So, too, is the flock of political sycophants who, shortly after the Capitol siege, condemned him and are now pledging their allegiance.

As for the third danger I had identified in that initial (2017) talk, finally, I called it *narrative solipsism*. And here I was referring to

> the kind of dynamic wherein narrative loses its foothold in the real and becomes hermetically self-enclosed, such that one comes to live in a storyworld of one's own making. That Donald Trump may be in the process of living in such a world is troubling in its own right. That others,

many others, seem to be joining him renders the situation nothing short of explosive. With these preliminary ideas in mind, let me offer a thesis of sorts: *When the relationship of narrative to reality is severed, we run the risk of falling prey to tyranny, the totalizing story being but a short step from totalitarianism.*

Suffice it to say, this concern remains. In fact, it is much more pronounced now, and much more troubling than it was then. Is it too much of a stretch to portray the current situation in these terms? I don't think so. And neither do many others (e.g., Levitsky & Ziblatt, 2019; Stanley, 2018). It should be noted that the dynamic being considered here is in no way limited to the United States. Nor, for that matter, is it limited to the present moment. Indeed, narrative solipsism—which is to say, the hermetic de-realization of reality itself in and through narrative—is, arguably, intrinsic to authoritarian politics (McIntyre, 2018) as well as a cornerstone of fascist thought and propaganda (Stanley, 2018).

The Intensification of the Threat

I do not mean to suggest that I was somehow prophetic in framing things the way I did back in 2017. Some of what I was seeing at the time was as clear as day, and plenty of others saw it. But little did I know just how bad and how scary things would get. I will call this second phase the *downright scary* phase. Consider for a moment some ideas put forth by Michiko Kakutani in her (2018) book *The Death of Truth: Notes on Falsehood in the Age of Trump*. After drawing some connections between Trump and certain strands of Bolshevism, Nazism, and so on, she goes on to suggest a connection between Trump and Putin, the latter's model of propaganda having been deemed " 'the firehose of falsehood'—an unremitting, high-intensity stream of lies, partial truths, and complete fictions spewed forth with tireless aggression to obfuscate the truth and overwhelm and confuse anyone trying to pay attention" (p. 141). Trump has made use of much the same sort of strategy, both during his term and after.

"The sheer volume of *desinformatsiya* unleashed by the Russian firehose system," Kakutani (2018) continues,

much like the more improvised but equally voluminous stream of lies, scandals, and shocks emitted by Trump, his GOP enablers, and media apparatchiks—tends to overwhelm and numb people while simultaneously defining deviancy down and normalizing the unacceptable. Outrage gives way to outrage fatigue, which gives way to the sort of cynicism and weariness that empowers those disseminating the lies. (p. 142)

Alongside the cacophony and the resultant confusion, there may be a shutting-out or a shutting-off, a reclusive sense of despair. Some people stop watching the news. Some turn to other things. Long walks outside. Bicycling. Bourbon. Occasionally, we are roused from this confusion and exhaustion and see a ray of light. "This time," we sometimes say, in the face of the latest instance of corruption, "is going to do it." People are going to wake up and see reality. *Finally.* The breaking point. Well, these "this times" have happened repeatedly. And narrative is partly to blame.

As CNN's Brian Stelter (2018) argued some time ago,

President Trump is winning the story-telling game, with help from his friends in the media. . . . Watch enough of [his] rallies, and his power as a storyteller shines through. He's the hero, the savior, the dragon-slayer of his own story. The villains include Democrats, foreigners and the journalists in the back of the hall. Love him or hate him, but give credit where it's due: Trump is succeeding at telling a story. Trump's stories are often more fiction than fact. But the thing about a story, like a novel or a drama, is that it's not really meant to be fact-checked. The narrative is meant to make you *feel.*

The apocalyticism idea is relevant in this context, too. "It's us versus them," Stelter writes, "darkness versus light." Lies abound. But many of them

are in service of the grand story he's telling. Look past the lies for a moment, and you can see why his crowds love it. He says he's putting America first, fixing the economy, and fighting the dark forces trying to stop him. His story is about wall-building and swamp-draining and deep-state-defeating.

And "he is the hero," while the "pro-Trump media act as his co-producers. . . . In Hollywood terms, it's as if Trump has a well-stocked writers room, where loyalists develop the plotlines for the next episodes." Stelter's concluding words:

In the same way that Disney fans fly to Florida, in the same way, that comic book fans argue on internet forums, Trump loyalists flock to his rallies. They are not representative of the public at large, but they do represent something powerful. They are motivated to defend him. And they're motivated to keep telling his story.

Lies and all.

This brings me back to the story I told about my daughter. A few years ago, at the biannual Psychology and the Other conference, I attended a session titled "Fascist Experience in a Traumatized World: The Embodiment of Us and Them." It wasn't just addressing Trump. Nor was it just addressing his followers. Rather, it was addressing all of us. At its foundation were two fundamental premises. First, no charismatic leader could mobilize the masses without their readiness. Second, we all contain elements of fascism, psychologically conceived, within us. And it's embodied most visibly in the us-versus-them dynamic. Again, this may be stretching the idea of fascism a bit too far, but it's provocative nonetheless and very much worth thinking about. This is another piece of the narrative puzzle and was masterfully and cruelly employed by Trump through blaming, scapegoating, and demonizing the feared and dreaded Other—immigrants, Democrats, scientists, inspectors general, Obama, China, all of whom were seen, in one way or another, to pose a threat, one thought to diminish and undermine one's own place in the world. *Them. They* did it. This part of the picture is no doubt familiar to many. But what also happens, and what may be somewhat less familiar, is that we who are constituted as the Them become reified into another Us, such that *they* become demonized, blanketed by our own modes of othering—which, I hate to admit, can be as narratively resistant and recalcitrant as that which we deplore. I am not about to get all lovey-dovey about this. I can't; the issues go too deep. Nor do I want to overrelativize things or establish some sort of spurious moral equivalence between us and them. Instead, I want to think about all this more, carefully and candidly and, if possible, compassionately, in the hope that it might ultimately lead me and others of my kind—as well as Them—beyond the despair and hostility and rage We (capital W) often feel. In any case, this second phase was indeed downright scary.

What Next?!

And then there was the emergence of the coronavirus. This is the phase we were in at the time of the Psychology of Global Crises conference. I will call this one the *narrative anxiety redoubled* phase. Lots of people in the States were anxious well before COVID-19 hit. "Narrative anxiety," you may recall, was something I mentioned earlier, in conjunction with the talk I gave in 2017 at the American University of Paris. This anxiety—and fear—has continued apace since that time, gaining strength all the while. How would it all play out? Many wondered. What does the future hold for us—and for democracy? There were lots of other things happening across the globe that added to this anxiety—politically, environmentally, technologically, and more—leading to a kind of existential anxiety born out of the sheer relentlessness of things. In some ways, I am talking here about the anxiety of narrative itself, the anxiety of not knowing the plot—or the ending—of the story-in-the-making being lived. So it is that history, Paul Ricoeur (1973) has written, may appear "as a play," but "with players who do not know the plot" (p. 102). To a greater or lesser extent, of course, it is always this way; there is a very real sense in which we never quite know what is going on until later on, in hindsight (Freeman, 2010). This is the ordinary anxiety of everyday life, in its indeterminacy and uncertainty. And it was certainly magnified by all the nonsense that had been going on for three years. Good God, many said, *What's next?!*

Well, now we know: *the coronavirus.* And with it, we have a number of new forms, or modes, of anxiety tied to new dimensions of indeterminacy and uncertainty. There is the anxiety of the virus itself. How bad is it? Am I going to get it? If I do, will I be asymptomatic, or will I be lying in bed hooked up to a ventilator, without family or friends, in misery? Will there be another variant? For those suffering from long COVID (i.e., those who have lingering and often debilitating symptoms following their bout with COVID), this anxiety may be magnified exponentially. Will my symptoms ever go away? Do I have a neurodegenerative disease? *What's happening to me?* Physicians still don't know. And that makes things even more painful for many.

There is the anxiety that's a function of the bizarre stew of information, misinformation, and disinformation and of not knowing the distribution of the three. Who do I believe? Who *can* I believe? And how is it possible, given what we *do* know, that some people, again, are flagrantly disregarding this knowledge? Do they really think they're invulnerable or that this is some hoax perpetrated by the deep state?

There is the anxiety of knowing, or at least suspecting, that other people are controlling and manipulating the narrative without quite knowing how or toward what end.

And, not least, there's the anxiety, and fear, of death, ubiquitous and visible as it has come to be, especially in the United States, where the death toll is approaching 1 million (CDC, 2022).

So, we are talking here about a multifaceted, multidimensional anxiety, a veritable perfect storm of anxiety, felt in varying degrees on the part of individuals, but lived, in one way or another, by all, even if on an unconscious plane. This anxiety is coupled with a sense of vulnerability, fragility, and loss for many—"the grieving of our assumptions," as Roger Frie put it in his talk at the conference, and, I would add, the grieving of the *life* that had existed before. And, of course, the grieving of the dead. The potentially positive side of this situation is the possibility of people acknowledging and accepting their vulnerability, perhaps leading to a kind of softening of selfhood, especially in its more hyper-agentic forms. Jens Brockmeier talked about this, too, on a more theoretical and disciplinary level, in an interesting and compelling way when he called for new, more decentered forms of theorizing the self.

But, of course, the consequences at hand aren't all positive. Yes, there may be posttraumatic growth for some. There may be moral and spiritual deepening, too, and a reimagining of life priorities. It is important to know this, to be sure. But there can also be quite severe negative consequences. And for those who had mental health difficulties before the virus came their way, the consequences might be that much more severe and that much more disabling. *Scary.* And, again, extremely dangerous. The reason is that this state of multifaceted and multidimensional anxiety and fear that we have been witnessing and experiencing has created a vacuum—a *vulnerability vacuum*, as we might call it—which often has, as its correlate, a receptivity and a susceptibility to those narratives, whether real or fictional, that promise some measure of deliverance from this very anxiety and fear. Trump and his cronies have sought to tap into this vacuum and are still in the process of doing exactly that. They have been engaged in a kind of psychological surveillance, as it were, seeing what veins of anxiety they can tap to bring some more followers on board. As I put the matter at the conference,

> There is no better way to do this, it seems than to offer up the promise not only of control but power and domination and liberation from those who threaten them and their way of life—even if it means violence.
>
> Aren't you hurting? Do you want to lose your livelihood—or your manhood? And aren't you getting frustrated by being locked up like a caged animal, all in the name of some allegedly pernicious threat that may not

even *be* one? Time to get back to it! "Liberate!" Trump told those gun- and rifle-toting protestors [in Michigan] who felt their cherished freedom was being undermined by being responsible to others. Regain control, agency, *pride*. "We will transition into greatness," Trump said recently. But that can only happen if you're freed from your cages. This means seeking and recruiting—sucking into the aforementioned vulnerability vacuum—all of those wayward, rudderless souls out there, many of them feeling *shame* and desperate to regain a sense of power and potency and make them a part of the winning team. It also means pitting people against one another and giving would-be zealots images and symbols that might serve to flame their fear and indignation and resentment of all who might interfere with their livelihood or their well-being. Don't blame me, Trump has said; I did nothing wrong. So, take all that hot emotion and project it onto others. I'll tell you who they are. Sprinkle it with absurd conspiracy theories. More demonization, more othering. If you don't join the team, the great American dream will go down the drain and you with it. It's an alluring narrative to many, and it's powerful—and it's no doubt endangering their health and, even perhaps, their very survival. That's what's happening now.

Not too long after I uttered those words, the Capitol siege happened. Again, I don't wish to claim prophecy. But once it was clear that Trump lost, that siege, or something like it, seemed all but inevitable. Narrative—the narrative of broken voting machines, the narrative of dead people voting, the theft, the hoax, the lie—played a large role in the process.

I went on in my conference talk to recount a headline I had read in the newspaper that morning: "Health officials warn weekend revelers of tragic impact." "It's an awful situation," I said.

The last thing anyone would want would be for this sort of thing to happen. This is no time for "I told you so's" or for saying "*Now* what do you think about your cherished freedom?" Don't go there; it's immoral and wrong. But the fact is, the statistics, terrible and terrifying as they are, haven't seemed to really "take" for lots of people; they're too abstract, too unfathomable. So here's another thought, one that brings us back to narrative and its allure and disturbing in its own right. In regard to the immigrant situation I referred to earlier, there seemed to be nothing that could budge people from the invasion-and-fear narrative until they heard stories, or saw images of children, crying and sometimes dying, in the hot sand and dirt of Texas or Arizona. Well, it may be that the only way to counter the triumphalist Trump-inspired narrative of prevailing over the pandemic, with its image of returning to life as we knew it, with our crowded restaurants and bars and football games, is by its inverted images. Not unlike the images of those crying and dying children, that means images and stories, of despair and death—the *faces*, as Emmanuel Levinas (e.g., 1985) might put it, of others, of flesh and blood *people*—that might be powerful enough to break through the crust of ideology or fantasy or willed ignorance, that can call us out of ourselves, that demand our attention and care. This is a horrible thought, truly. I hope and pray that we don't get to that point.

In fact, I hope I'm wrong about the picture I've been painting here. But the fact is, we, in the States, are witnessing a narrative about making America great again that is so ideologically rooted and so consistently and ruthlessly fueled by a barrage of information, misinformation, and disinformation that it seems utterly immoveable, utterly resistant to any new episode of vileness or stupidity or mendacity that might, in some other world, change the course of things. As I've already suggested, it's very scary and very dangerous. That the coronavirus pandemic is a global crisis has become a truism. But it might be suggested, cautiously of course, that the more dangerous pandemic may be found in those various movements, in the United States and elsewhere, that involve the full-on spread of misinformation and disinformation and, in turn, the full-scale misshaping and corruption and de-realization of reality itself. A *narrative* pandemic, as it were. Unfortunately, there's no vaccine for it. Not now, not ever. (Freeman, 2020)

I *was* wrong about that picture I painted. The fact is, there have been plenty of images and stories of despair and death. But they haven't broken through that "crust" I had referred to, "the crust of ideology or fantasy or willed ignorance." The narratives at hand are too entrenched, too immoveable, too resistant to reality.

Consider a headline from *The Washington Post* (February 5, 2022) I came across: "The Republican Party formally declares that truth is fiction and patriots are traitors." As the piece goes on to state, "The Orwellian censure resolution accuses Ms. Cheney and fellow GOP dissident Rep. Adam Kinzinger (R-Ill.) of engaging in behavior 'destructive to the institution of the U.S. House of Representatives, the Republican Party and our republic'" by serving on the committee investigating the Capitol siege. Why? That investigation, according to the resolution, is nothing more than " 'a Democrat-led

persecution of ordinary citizens engaged in legitimate political discourse.'"
Wow. Let's get real, the editorial continues,

> Republicans assailing Ms. Cheney and siding with Mr. Trump and his lies
> about the 2020 election are the ones who imperil the republic. By asserting,
> as their censure resolution did Friday, that truth is fiction and patriots are
> turncoats, they have exposed the dark, festering core of what their party is
> becoming: an unruly revolt against fact and reason.

As scary as things were at the time of the conference, they are scarier
now. Much.

Looking Toward the Future

I concluded the 2020 conference talk by offering what I called a "triple hermeneutic." In doing so, I said the following:

> First, in line with the more positive pictures painted by others, there's the
> need for a *hermeneutics of hope*, or faith. This hope is not only for individual
> flourishing but also for the larger, more macro societal restructuring and
> environmental repair that are so sorely needed, in the States and elsewhere.
> Many people at this conference have made a compelling case for this.
>
> Second, there's the need for a *hermeneutics of vigilance*, or suspicion, cri-
> tique, one that remains attuned to the allure of narrative and, more gener-
> ally, the instrumental machinations and diversionary tactics of those who
> would privilege their own political ends over the health and well-being of
> suffering and oppressed people. I mean this in relation to both the current
> pandemic and the larger one I referred to a little while back.
>
> Third, and finally, there's the need for a *hermeneutics of compas-
> sion*, oriented not only toward the suffering and oppressed people I just
> mentioned but also toward those others, those "Thems," we might despise.
> Ideally, this would lead not to the much vaunted "return to normal" many
> seek; that normal wasn't so great for lots of people. Instead, it would lead
> to a new, more capacious solidarity, one that would welcome the stranger,
> even the feared or dreaded or despised other, into its midst. Easier said than
> done, I know. And truthfully, I don't think I'll be able to do it with Trump
> or McConnell. *Ever.* But without this hermeneutics of compassion, without

some image of shared humanity, we'll surely be led into still more troubled waters.

It's hard for me to read these words now. I suppose there is always room for hope. But given that COVID-related deaths continue to pile up, almost exclusively among the unvaccinated, and given stories like the one I just shared about Liz Cheney and Adam Kinzinger, I can't say I have much of it.

Regarding the second element, vigilance, I am certainly still committed to that, but, if truth be told, I am not sure how much it matters. Much of what we are witnessing doesn't even require vigilance; it's perfectly clear. People are being lured by narrative to their untimely deaths. Politicians are being lured by narrative to flaunt reality altogether and are leading the United States down a dark, dangerous, and potentially deadly path.

As for the hermeneutics of compassion, well, I am still finding that difficult to practice. I wish it wasn't so. Many of the people carrying ignorance and violence forward are victims of narrative, lured by opportunists of one stripe or another seeking power. I do feel for some of them—especially those who, on their death bed or sitting bedside next to a loved one, grieve over what they wouldn't, and couldn't, see owing to the power of the storylines that came their way. In the case others, it's more of a challenge to summon up this sympathy and compassion. I also cannot help but wonder: What really is called for at this particular moment? Empathy, understanding, and compassion? Righteous indignation? Fighting fire with fire by digging into our own bag of narrative tricks, in the hope that We might tell stories that are as alluring as Theirs? I really don't know; we are too much *in medias res*—in the middle—to know how to move forward. I just hope that we don't look backward at some point in the future and say: "We knew what was happening, and we ought to have done more to stop it." As always, time will tell.

References

CDC. (2022). https://www.cdc.gov/coronavirus/2019-ncov/covid-data/covidview/index.html

Freeman, M. (2010). *Hindsight: The promise and peril of looking backward*. Oxford University Press.

Freeman, M. (2014). *The priority of the Other: Thinking and living beyond the self*. Oxford University Press.

Freeman, M. (2017). Whose story? Whose world? Life and narrative in the age of Trump. Lecture presented at the American University of Paris, Paris, France.

Freeman, M. (2020). The (Al)lure of narrative: Information, misinformation, and dis-information in the time of coronavirus. Lecture presented at virtual conference on "The Psychology of Global Crises: State Surveillance, Solidarity, and Everyday Life," American University of Paris, Paris, France.

Freud, S. (1962). Civilization and its discontents. *Standard Edition XXI*. Hogarth. (Original work published 1930.)

Kakutani, M. (2018). *The death of truth: Notes on falsehood in the age of Trump*. Tim Duggan Books.

Levi, P. (1989). *The drowned and the saved*. Vintage.

Levinas, E. (1985). *Ethics and infinity*. Duquesne University Press.

Levitsky, S., & Ziblatt, D. (2019). *How democracies die*. Crown.

McIntyre, L. (2018). *Post-truth*. MIT Press.

Ricoeur, P. (1973). The model of the text: Meaningful action considered as a text. *New Literary History, 5*, 91–117.

Stanley, J. (2018). *How fascism works: The politics of us and them*. Random House.

Stelter, B. (2018). President Trump is winning the storytelling game, with help from his friends in the media. https://money.cnn.com/2018/08/05/media/donald-trump-story-telling/index.html

Trump, D. (2017). Presidential inauguration speech. https://www.politico.eu/article/this-american-carnage-stops-right-here/amp/

Turner, V. (1995). *The ritual process: Structure and anti-structure*. Routledge.

Washington Post. (2022). https://www.washingtonpost.com/opinions/2022/02/04/liz-cheney-republicans-censure-orwellian/

3

Stories of Crisis

Denial, Redemption, and Radical Acceptance in the Time of COVID-19

Dan P. McAdams

In his celebrated novel, *The Plague*, Albert Camus (1947) tells the story of a virus spreading uncontrollably through a small city on the Algerian coast. For almost a year, the citizens are locked down and cut off from the rest of the world as the epidemic claims thousands of lives. The pestilence brings tremendous suffering and unremitting uncertainty. It is impossible to predict who will survive the onslaught of the pathogen and who will succumb. Moreover, nobody knows when, and even if, the crisis will end. Different characters in the novel offer their own interpretations of the epidemic. In their efforts to make meaning amid the carnage, they tell stories.

The COVID-19 pandemic of 2020–2022 brought untold suffering to millions of human beings across the globe and unremitting uncertainty. As I write these words in January of 2022, approximately two years after the virus was identified in Wuhan, China, well over 5 million people worldwide have died from the pandemic. Nearly a fifth of those deaths (nearing 900,000) have occurred in the United States. For many nations, the economic effects have been devastating. In 2021, new and deadlier variants of the virus emerged after many people felt the worse was over. The good news in 2021, however, was that effective vaccines were developed and disseminated, though wealthier nations generally enjoyed much easier access to vaccines than did the Global South. Toward the end of 2021, the Omicron variant emerged. Rabidly contagious but producing significantly less severe illness, Omicron led to both dread and hope—dread regarding the renewed strain on health-care systems with the rapid rise of new cases and hope that the surprisingly mild symptoms that usually (though not always) resulted, combined with the dissemination of effective vaccines and boosters, might ultimately lead to a

Dan P. McAdams, *Stories of Crisis* In: *Narrative in Crisis*. Edited by: Martin Dege and Irene Strasser,
Oxford University Press. © Oxford University Press 2024. DOI: 10.1093/oso/9780197751756.003.0003

new and manageable normal. Then again, the virus has proved remarkably unpredictable, so the future is uncertain.

In ways all too familiar to the fictional characters in *The Plague*, people living during the time of COVID-19 create stories to comprehend the pandemic, its effects on their own lives, and its meaning for the world in general. Ever since human beings invented language, and perhaps even before, we have made sense of experience through narrative (Dor, 2015; McAdams & Cowan, 2021). Usually conveyed in words and images, but also through the body's movements and other performative modes, stories create meaning by framing intentional human action within the contexts of consciousness and temporality (Bruner, 1986; Ricoeur, 1984). Stories track transformation in the thoughts and feelings of goal-directed agents as they move across time. They convey what characters want, how they pursue what they want, and aim to avoid what they do not want, from one scene to the next, from beginning through middle to end. People tell stories about individual moments in their lives, about their lives as a whole, about their families and their communities as they have evolved over time, and about history. As a world-historic event, the COVID-19 pandemic has impacted families and communities the world over, shaped the course of individual human lives, and infiltrated daily quotidian events. From the sweep of history to the meaning of yesterday afternoon's interaction with a masked stranger, what stories might people construct to make sense of the pandemic in the time of COVID-19?

Drawing from research and theory on narrative identity (McAdams & McLean, 2013) as articulated within the fields of personality and life span developmental psychology, I propose three different kinds of stories that may be invoked to make meaning out of the pandemic. In a nutshell, they are stories of (1) denial, (2) redemption, and (3) radical acceptance. In each form, the virus itself becomes a character in the story. In stories of denial, the virus is a malevolent but ephemeral force whose actions and effects are limited to a discrete moment in time. In stories of redemption, the virus is a more persistent adversary who will be defeated in the long run, to the benefit of the victors. In stories of radical acceptance, the virus never fully goes away but represents instead an enduring nemesis who must be managed within a narrative that bears honest witness to human suffering.

Who are the storytellers for the three narrative forms I am about to describe? The answer is pretty much *anybody*. The forms may be manifest in media accounts of the pandemic, in the ways politicians and policymakers frame the pandemic in public discourse, and how everyday people, including survivors of the illness, make sense of their lives in the time of pandemic and how they imagine the future (Greene, 2021). Each of the three forms is elastic enough to fit the needs of a wide range of storytellers. That said, there is no claim of universality here. There are surely many other ways to make narrative sense of the COVID-19 pandemic. Moreover, cultural norms and local circumstances are always prime factors in determining how people talk about their lived experience, putting limits on how confident any scholar can be in identifying broad and generalizable forms. Operating in the context of discovery, I offer these three forms as an opening suggestion, hoping to stimulate thinking about the different kinds of stories people may tell about life in the time of COVID-19.

A Moment in Time

As developed from McAdams's (1985) life story model of identity, the concept of *narrative identity* refers to people's internalized and evolving self-stories that explain how they have come to be the persons they are becoming (McAdams & McLean, 2013). Combining the selective reconstruction of the past with a person's imagined future, narrative identity includes the main chapters (past and future) that people identify in their lives, key self-defining scenes such as personal high points and low points, important characters that have influenced the course of events, and the general themes and through-lines that characterize how people make sense of their own lives in time.

An important feature of narrative identity is *autobiographical reasoning*, which is the broad conclusions or lessons that people draw about their lives and identities based on the specific autobiographical material that they recall and narrate to others (Habermas & Bluck, 2000; McLean et al., 2007). When engaging in autobiographical reasoning, people typically process the concrete specifics in their lives, including especially negative events, in order to arrive at broader meanings about who they are and what their lives may signify. But narrators exhibit large individual differences in the extent to which they tend to engage in autobiographical reasoning (Hallford & Mellor, 2017). Whereas some people readily derive deep meanings and broad themes in narrating events in their lives, others find very little meaning at all (Strawson, 2004). What may sound like a life-changing or self-defining event as told by one narrator may hold little or no meaning as told by another. In the latter case, the narrator may suggest something like this: "It happened. It's over. Let's move on."

People who engage in very little autobiographical reasoning tend to see their lives in *episodic* terms. Rather than linking scenes together and deriving integrative thematic meanings in their lives, they tend instead to focus on the particulars of each discrete episode. Even when research interviewers encourage them to expand on the meanings of events in their lives, people with an episodic approach to life narration resist the demand. They may even express impatience or annoyance when repeatedly asked to probe beneath the surface in life narration. In one interview study, researchers determined that approximately 5% of respondents showed a strongly episodic approach to life narration (Turner et al., 2020). Interestingly, this small group did not appear to differ systematically from the other participants on any of a range of self-report psychological measures administered in this study. Unlike the vast majority of the other respondents, however, this small group did not experience substantial increases in positive emotion over the course of the session, as determined by mood scales administered immediately before and after being interviewed. They did not find the process of telling their life stories to be especially engaging. When explicitly asked to consider the meanings of particular events in their lives, they repeatedly refused to engage in autobiographical reasoning. It was not clear if their refusals were due to an inability to make meaning out of life events or a motivated desire not to do so.

The findings from Turner et al. (2020) dovetail with an in-depth case study I conducted on the life and personality of Donald J. Trump, the 45th president of the United States (McAdams, 2020). In *The strange case of Donald J. Trump: A psychological reckoning*, I drew upon well-established empirical findings in personality and developmental science, as well as evidence-based theories, to make psychological sense of Trump's life and his presidency. The book's central thesis is that Trump is the quintessential *episodic man*, living outside of time and narrative, immersed forever in the combative moment. The many notable features of his personality—from his malignant narcissism to his authoritarian sentiments to his dynamic, charismatic traits—revolve around an empty core, like a vortex. In the middle, where the story should be but never was, is a narrative vacuum. Donald Trump has no story in his mind about who he is and how he came to be, no story of change and development. He simply is and has always been—fully formed Trump, a "stable genius," to use an expression he has applied without irony to himself, as if sprung full-form from the head of Zeus. Trump's philosophy of life, as told in an interview with *People* magazine more than 40 years ago, is this: "Man is the most vicious of all animals, and life is a series of battles ending in victory or defeat" (D'Antonio, 2015, p. 154). What he meant is that each battle itself ends in victory or defeat. One after another. The only goal is to win the battle you are in right now—today, in the current episode. And then move on to the next.

How might a person who sees life in purely episodic terms make sense of the coronavirus? It was a huge challenge for President Trump in 2020, because the virus is part of a long-term story and Trump lives in the current moment. On March 11, 2020, Trump characterized the problem of the virus as confined to a "temporary moment in time" (Blake & Rieger, 2020). Two weeks before then, he predicted that the virus would be here today, gone tomorrow: "One day it's like a miracle, it will disappear" (Blake & Rieger, 2020). On certain days in January and February of 2020, he denied that the virus even existed. It was all a plot hatched by his enemies to bring down his presidency. On other days, he conceded that there was a virus but that the United States was uniquely safe, as if the nation existed outside the bounds of time and space. Moving through his presidency moment by discrete moment, each moment separated from what came before and what may follow, fighting to win each moment in time, Donald Trump repeatedly stated or did whatever he felt to be necessary to win what he perceived to be the battle of the moment. One day he urged Americans to rise up against their state's governors and force businesses to reopen during the pandemic. The very next day, he criticized a state's governor for doing exactly what he told the protestors to do. When it felt right in the moment, he claimed that an unproved drug was a miracle cure for COVID-19. On another occasion in April of 2020, he entertained the idea that sick people might be injected with bleach.

Because he lives outside the narrative flow of time, Trump was psychologically unable to articulate a long-term plan to address the pandemic, and he was unable to support the development of such a plan. He was unable to formulate a plausible narrative that extends back into the past and forward into the distant future to explain what has happened and what the American people might do, step by step, to alter the plot and move the story in a better direction, to flatten the curve of infections, for example, to arrive at something that looks like a better place after a long and difficult journey. Instead, he thinks about the situation the way many of the citizens in the Algerian town thought about the plague in its early days. Camus (1947) wrote of sensing "a void within which never left us, that irrational longing to hark back to the past or else speed up the march of time" (p. 65). In other words, let us magically make the present moment like it was yesterday or fast-forward to the day the virus disappears. In sum, then, President Trump's narrative for the pandemic went something like this: *The virus will go away—I know it will! And then we will get back to where we were. And we will be great again.*

While Trump's refusal to take the virus seriously—his refusal to make meaning of the virus in time—has been resoundingly criticized, it should be noted that denial is sometimes a good thing. And there may be value, under certain conditions, of apprehending reality in episodic terms. Psychological research amply demonstrates that some people cope best with severe adversity by simply brushing it off. In a highly influential formulation, Bonanno (2004) has shown that many people experience surprisingly little angst and turmoil when stricken with harsh misfortunes in life. Their resilience is rooted in denial. Mark Freeman (2011a, 2011b) has argued that some traumatic and especially shameful experiences in life cannot be readily incorporated into narrative identity because the narrator (and perhaps the people to whom the narrator might tell the story) lacks the world assumptions, cognitive constructs, or experiential categories to make the story make sense. Memories of these kinds of events, therefore, may be buried in what Freeman describes as a *narrative unconscious.*

For some people in some circumstances, it may be psychologically best to resist meaning-making and simply go on with life. Research on trauma suggests that denial can be an effective coping mechanism, especially early in a recovery process (Altmaeir, 2017). Random acts of violence or destruction may prove too painful to revisit, too emotionally difficult to assimilate into one's life story. Donald Trump's dismissal of the virus as nothing more than a moment in time may be extreme in the extent to which the president failed to take the pandemic seriously. Nonetheless, under conditions of crisis, many people may find some psychological solace in stories of denial, as did presumably some of the citizens in Camus's fictional town.

Redemptive Stories

In stories of redemption, the protagonist is delivered from suffering through a positive turn of events or through a retrospective reframing emphasizing growth, recovery, liberation, or some other positive psychological meaning (McAdams, 2013). A negative life event is salvaged, redeemed, or transformed by a positive outcome or meaning. From the realm of clinical psychology, one of the best examples of such a transformation is the phenomenon of *posttraumatic growth* (Tedeschi & Calhoun, 2004).

Survivors of combat, natural disasters, physical abuse, and other traumatic experiences sometimes report later that they gained an unexpected benefit from the horrific event. Without downplaying the suffering, they may report that their negative experience gave them a new insight about their lives, or taught them to cherish life more, or brought them closer to the people they love, or closer to God. They feel that they experienced some form of personal growth as a result of the trauma (Altmaeir, 2017).

Research in many different subfields of psychology shows that people often strive to make positive meaning out of negative events—little ones and big ones. The research also suggests that people who are more or less successful in creating redemptive stories in the wake of negative events tend to enjoy higher levels of mental health and psychological well-being (Adler et al., 2015; Dunlop & Tracy, 2013; McAdams et al., 2001).

Notable in this regard is research into the life stories told by highly *generative* midlife American adults. As described first by Erik Erikson (1963), to be generative in midlife is to commit oneself to the well-being and development of future generations. Parenting is the quintessential arena wherein generativity is expressed. But generativity is also expressed in teaching, mentoring, civic engagement, leadership, and a range of other behaviors and commitments aimed at leaving a positive legacy of the self for future generations.

How do highly generative adults narrate their lives? Findings from many studies, both quantitative (McAdams & Guo, 2015) and qualitative (McAdams, 2013), show that highly generative adults are more likely than their less generative counterparts to construct redemptive stories to make sense of their lives. Their stories converge on a general narrative form, articulated through five general themes and called *the redemptive self* (McAdams, 2013). In the paradigmatic story of the redemptive self, the protagonist learns early in life that (1) they are special or blessed and (2) the world is a dangerous place where many people suffer. Equipped with (3) steadfast moral values, the protagonist encounters many failures and setbacks in life, but these are often (4) redeemed by positive outcomes or meanings. Looking to the future, the protagonist (5) hopes to continue to promote the well-being of others and leave a positive legacy.

Redemptive stories affirm hope and a commitment to making the world a better place. Creating a narrative identity that features many scenes wherein bad things lead to good outcomes may sustain the optimism and faith people need to persevere in the face of adversity. The juxtaposition of early advantage and the suffering of others—the sense that I am special and that the world needs me—may motivate prosocial behavior and provide a narrative frame for making sense of altruism and civic responsibility. There is often a sense of gratitude in redemptive life stories as told by highly generative American adults. I have been fortunate in my life, the story says. And I need to give back.

It is easy to see how redemptive narratives might help people to make sense of and cope with the coronavirus crisis. We will get through this, the story says. There will be tremendous suffering, but, in the long run, we will emerge stronger for what we went through. In a *New York Times* column, David Brooks (2020) expressed the hope that Americans will find long-term redemptive meaning in the virus. "We will look back on this as one of the most meaningful periods of our lives," Brooks (2020) wrote. Our long-term well-being depends on "the story we tell about this moment. It's the way we tie our moment of suffering to a larger narrative of redemption. It's the way we then go out and stubbornly live out that story. The plague today is an invisible monster, but it gives birth to a better world."

In the early days of the pandemic, not a day went by on social media, on television, in the newspapers without the proliferation of redemptive stories about the coronavirus. Some of these were dramatic stories of recovery, starring nurses and first-responders who minister to the victims, and starring those victims themselves, of course, who, after weeks on a respirator, manage to come back from the precipice. Others are narratives that find unexpected benefits in the shutdowns, with the hope that a new era will usher in a more prosperous, peaceful, or verdant world. In April of 2020, the New Zealand-born poet Tomos Roberts (aka TomFoolery) uploaded a video to YouTube that told an especially redemptive story of the virus. A young father is telling his son a bedtime story entitled "The Great Realisation": "It was a world of waste and wonder / of poverty and plenty / back before we understood / why hindsight's 2020." Set in an idyllic post-COVID future, the story looks back in hindsight to a dystopian era—that is, the years before 2020—when the world was starkly divided between the rich and the poor, when people lost themselves in their smartphones, as the planet burned. The 4-minute video suggests humankind must have gotten through it all, traveled the long redemptive passage to a better world. Still, when the story ends, the little boy wants to know: "Why did it take a virus to bring the people together?"

Radical Acceptance

In Camus's *The Plague*, it is not clear that the pathogen *did* "bring the people together." After months and months of mounting deaths, the narrator remarks that the Algerian citizens were living "without memories, without hope." "There is no denying that the plague had gradually killed off in all of us the faculty not of love only but even of friendship" (Camus, 1947, p. 165). Thankfully, the citizens do get through it all, the survivors, that is, and there is something like a happy ending to the story. Almost a year into the epidemic, the pathogen seems to wear out. Perhaps the town has achieved herd immunity or the virus mutates into a less toxic variant. For whatever reason, victims begin to recover. A young girl lying in a hospital bed, her prognosis deemed to be "hopeless," suddenly revives. The night before, she was "delirious and had all the symptoms of pneumonic plague," but the next morning "her temperature had fallen." She is now in the clear. The doctors observe that her recovery went "against all the rules" (Camus, 1947, pp. 239–240). The plague subsides. The city opens up. The citizens rejoice.

The story's narrator, however, cautions against a redemptive interpretation for *The Plague*: "The tale could not be one of a final victory," the narrator says. "It could be only the record of what had had to be done, and what assuredly would have to be done again in the never-ending fight against terror and its relentless onslaughts, despite their personal afflictions, by all who, while unable to be saints but refusing to bow down to pestilences, strive their utmost to be healers" (Camus, 1947, p. 278).

The central protagonist in *The Plague* is Dr. Benjamin Rieux. He is, we must assume, the model for "the healer" in stories of this kind. Along with a small group of friends and associates, Dr. Rieux ministers to the sick and dying during the many months when the pestilence ravages the city. He puts in 18-hour days, moving back and forth between hospital wards and victims' homes. It is grueling work. Yet Rieux insists that he is not a hero. "There's no question of heroism in all this," he tells a friend. "It's a matter of common decency. That's an idea that may make people smile," Rieux confesses, "but the only means of fighting a plague is common decency." His friend asks him: What does that mean? What is common decency? Rieux says: "I don't know what it means for other people. But in my case I know that it consists in doing my job" (Camus, 1947, p. 150).

Many readers point to the above passage as the key to understanding Camus's fundamental message. This is not a heart-warming story of redemption. *The Plague* is not centrally about a gifted, morally steadfast hero, a la the redemptive self, who sets off on a journey to transform the world. Instead, the hero is merely doing his job. Granted it is a very hard job and a noble one. Still, if we see his job as healing, then we have to admit that Dr. Rieux was mainly a failure. Camus documents very few, if any, instances in which Dr. Rieux actually saves a life. He doesn't really heal anybody. Having said that, Rieux is an extraordinarily admirable character. And there is something about the overall story told, even if it is not especially redemptive, that rings of compelling authenticity. Something clear-sighted and deeply humane.

What is the story being told here? It would seem to involve a *radical acceptance* of the world as it is coupled with the valiant effort to manage the uncertainty of that world. Radical acceptance should not be confused with resignation. The story is not about selling out and giving up and going along blithely with the status quo. On the pestilence, Dr. Rieux observes: "I know it's an absurd situation, but we're all involved in it, and we've got to accept it as it is" (Camus, 1947, p. 79). When one friend observes that the plague confronts the medical establishment with one "defeat" after another, Rieux says: "Yes, I know that. But it's no reason for giving up the struggle" (Camus, 1947, p. 118).

Theory and research on the psychological value of acceptance feature prominently in the literature on adult development and aging. For example, Erikson (1963) identified *ego integrity versus despair* to be the prime psychosocial challenge of the later years in life, as strivings for generativity begin to recede. According to Erikson, ego integrity involves a graceful acceptance of one's very life, whereas despair entails bitterness, rejection, and extensive regret. With respect to empirical work, life-narrative researchers have shown that midlife adults who score high on self-report measures of ego integrity tend to articulate life stories that renounce regret and display a good deal of *self-transcendence* (Reischer et al., 2020).

Different conceptions of *wisdom* converge on the idea that to be wise is, in part, to transcend egoistic strivings of the self in order to operate effectively in an ambiguous world wherein human beings face implacable limitations in what they can do and know (Baltes & Staudinger, 2000; Grossman, 2017). Therefore, wisdom entails intellectual humility, awareness of context, perspective flexibility, and the recognition of uncertainty and uncontrollable change in the world. To be wise is to accept gracefully and manage effectively the inherent uncertainty of human affairs. In support of this assertion, one study of adults ranging in age from 26 to 92 years found that wisdom was positively associated with a tendency to explore the nuances of difficult life experiences (Westrate & Glück, 2017). Rather than try to change life, wisdom lay in accepting it as something given—indeed, accepting suffering as part and parcel of being human, as if suffering itself were like an externalized object prompting reflection and examination. By contrast, the tendency to find redemptive meanings in difficult life experiences was unrelated to wisdom.

Working within a psychodynamic frame, Elliot Jacques (1965) observed that creative artists and musicians often discover a tragic and philosophical dimension of their work in the second half of life. The Israeli psychotherapists Nahi Alon and Haim Omer (2004) underscored the value of just such a perspective in counseling and therapy. In ancient Greek and Shakespearian tragedies, the hero learns that suffering is unavoidable in life and often irredeemable. Tragedy teaches that human beings cannot always control their own affairs (Doerries, 2015). Instead, fate, serendipity, and other capricious factors often prove the ultimate determinants of behavior and experience. These factors rarely produce simple happy endings in life but instead engender complexity and empathy. Alon and Omer (2004) insist that recognizing and accepting this fact can have profoundly salutary effects for many people. As an antidote to the heroic striving of the morally righteous redemptive self, tragic stories teach acceptance and humility while opening people up to each other and building bonds of intimacy.

In sum, building a life narrative around the idea of radical acceptance might work off of the following simple template. The story's setting is a world of uncertainty, unpredictable change, and serendipity—life in the time of COVID-19. The idealized goal in the story is to come to terms with life, reconcile conflicts to minimize regret, manage adversity (because adversity cannot always be overcome), and sustain bonds of intimacy and warmth. Dr. Rieux is the kind of protagonist who flourishes in this kind of story, manifestly expressing personal characteristics such as grace, humility, and flexibility.

Seven pages from the end of the novel, Camus gives the big reveal. He reports that the narrator of this story all along has been Dr. Rieux himself. Up to this point in the book, the reader thinks of Rieux as the protagonist who is doing his job as a doctor. But it turns out that Rieux is much more than that. His paramount role throughout the novel turns out *not* to have been treating the sick and dying during a time of plague. He did that, of course. But, more than that, Dr. Rieux, as narrator, *bears witness* to the plague. In his own words, his primary job—the job that required such a wealth of common decency—was "to be an honest witness." Camus writes: "Dr. Rieux resolved to compile this chronicle, so that he should not be one of those who hold their peace but should bear witness in favor of those plague-stricken people; so that some memorial of the injustice and outrage done them might endure; and to state quite simply what we learn in a time of pestilence: that there are more things to admire in men than to despise" (Camus, 1947, p. 278).

The *episodic* approach to life in the time of COVID-19 is to deny reality and hope for a magic return to what was. The *redemptive* approach anticipates that positive meanings will ultimately redeem our suffering. Dr. Rieux's message, as narrator and protagonist of a story of *radical acceptance*, is not as blithely optimistic as the message of redemption. Still, the story sustains hope. The story says that we must bear witness to the suffering of our fellow humans. We have to accept the suffering. We cannot look away. We have to be clear-eyed. Whether or not we are able to overcome adversity in our lives (and we should try to do so), we also have to learn to manage it and to accept the fact that it is likely to be with us always, in one form or another. We have to come to terms with the world as it is and to human beings as they are, rather than how we wish the world and people were.

In the last sentences of *The Plague*, Dr. Rieux reports that the city is now filled with joy. Happiness abounds after the plague, and Dr. Rieux celebrates with his fellow citizens. But Rieux knows that the joy will always be imperiled. Plagues and pestilences—and the infinite sources of human misery—will be with us always. That is *the story of life* in Rieux's narrating mind at the end of the time of the plague. Dr. Rieux wants us to know that the very same human story might apply across the board in many different times and places.

References

Adler, J. M., Brookshier, K., Monahan, C., Walder-Biesanz, I., Harmeling, L. H., Albaugh, M., McAdams, D. P., & Oltmanns, T. F. (2015). Variation in narrative identity isassociated with trajectories of mental health over several years. *Journal of Personality and Social Psychology, 108*, 476–496.

Alon, N., & Omer, H. (2004). Demonic and tragic narratives in psychotherapy. In A. Lieblich, D. P. McAdams, and R. Josselson (Eds.), *Healing plots: The narrative bases of psychotherapy* (pp. 29–48). Washington, DC: APA Books.

Altmaeir, B. (Ed.). (2017). *Meaning reconstruction after trauma*. London: Elsevier.

Baltes, P. B., & Staudinger, U. M. (2000). Wisdom: A metaheuristic (pragmatic) to orchestrate mind and virtue toward excellence. *American Psychologist, 55*, 122–136.

Blake, A., & Rieger, J. (2020, November 3). Timeline: The 201 times Trump has downplayed the coronavirus threat. *The Washington Post.* https://www.washingtonpost.com/politics/2020/03/12/trump-coronavirus-timeline/

Bonanno, G. (2004). Loss, trauma, and human resilience: Have we underestimatedthe human capacity to thrive after extremely adverse events? *American Psychologist, 59*, 20–28.

Brooks, D. (2020, March 26). The moral meaning of the plague. *New York Times.* https://www.nytimes.com/2020/03/26/opinion/coronavirus-meaning.html

Bruner, J. (1986). *Actual minds, possible worlds.* Harvard University Press.

Camus, A. (1947). *The plague.* New York: Knopf.

D'Antonio, M. (2015). *Never enough: Donald Trump and the pursuit of success.* St. Martin's Press.

Doerries, B. (2015). *The theater of war: What ancient Greek tragedies can teach us today.* Vintage.

Dor, D. (2015). *The instruction of imagination: Language as a social communication technology.* Oxford University Press.

Dunlop, W. L., & Tracy, J. L. (2013). Sobering stories: Narratives of self-redemption predict behavioral change and improved health among recovering alcoholics. *Journal of Personality and Social Psychology, 104*, 576–590.

Erikson, E. H. (1963). *Childhood and society* (2nd ed.). Norton.

Freeman, M. (2011a). Narrative foreclosure in later life: Possibilities and limits. In G. Kenyon, E. Bohlmeijer, & W. L. Randall (Eds.), *Storying later life: Issues, investigations, and interventions in narrative gerontology* (pp. 3–19). Oxford University Press.

Freeman, M. (2011b). The space of selfhood: Culture, narrative, identity. In S. R. Kirschner & J. Martin (Eds.), *The sociocultural turn in psychology: The contextual emergence of mind and self* (pp. 137–158). Columbia University Press.

Greene, M. F. (2021, May). You won't remember the pandemic the way you think you will. *The Atlantic*, 58–68.

Grossman, I. (2017). Wisdom in context. *Perspectives on Psychological Science, 12*, 233–257.

Habermas, T., & Bluck, S. (2000). Getting a life: The emergence of the life story in adolescence. *Psychological Bulletin, 126*, 748–769.

Hallford, D., & Mellor, D. (2017). Development and validation of the Awareness of Narrative Identity Questionnaire (ANIQ). *Assessment, 24*, 399–413.

Jacques, E. (1965). Death and the midlife crisis. *International Journal of Psycho-Analysis, 46*, 502–515.

McAdams, D. P. (1985). *Power, intimacy, and the life story: Personological inquiries into identity.* Guilford.

McAdams, D. P. (2013). *The redemptive self: Stories Americans live by* (revised and expanded edition). Oxford University Press.

McAdams, D. P. (2020). *The strange case of Donald J. Trump: A psychological reckoning.* Oxford University Press.

McAdams, D. P., & Cowan, R. (2021). Mimesis and myth: Evolutionary origins of psychological self-understanding. In J. Carroll (Ed.), *Evolutionary perspectives on imaginative culture* (pp. 93–108). Springer.

McAdams, D. P., & Guo, J. (2015). Narrating the generative life. *Psychological Science, 26*, 475–483.

McAdams, D. P., & McLean, K. C. (2013). Narrative identity. *Current Directions in Psychological Science, 22*, 233–238.

McAdams, D. P., Reynolds, J., Lewis, M., Patten, A., & Bowman, P. J. (2001). When bad things turn good and good things turn bad: Sequences of redemption and contamination in life narrative, and their relation to psychosocial adaptation in midlife adults and in students. *Personality and Social Psychology Bulletin, 27*, 472–483.

McLean, K. C., Pasupathi, M., & Pals, J. (2007). Selves creating stories creating selves: A process model of self-development. *Personality and Social Psychology Review, 11*, 262–278.

Reischer, H. N., Roth, L. J., Villarreal, J. A., & McAdams, D. P. (2020). Self-transcendence and life stories of humanistic growth among late-midlife adults. *Journal of Personality, 89*, 305–324.

Ricoeur, P. (1984). *Time and narrative* (vol. 1; K. McGlaughin and D. Pellauer, trans.). University of Chicago Press.

Strawson, G. (2004). Against narrativity. *Ratio, 17*, 428–451.

Tedeschi, R. G., & Calhoun, L. G. (2004). Posttraumatic growth: The conceptual foundations and empirical evidence. *Psychological Inquiry, 15*, 1–18.

Turner, A., Cowan, H. R., Otto-Meyer, R., & McAdams, D. P. (2020). The power of narrative: The emotional impact of the life story interview. *Narrative Inquiry*. https://doi.org/10.1075/ni.19109.tur

Westrate, N. M., & Glück, J. (2017). Hard-earned wisdom: Exploratory processing of difficult life experience is positively associated with wisdom. *Developmental Psychology, 53*, 800–814.

4

Dominant and Counteracting Narratives of "Crisis" in COVID Times

Corinne Squire

Introduction

Many early accounts of the COVID-19 pandemic described it as a "crisis": a dangerous, turning-point moment from which, as a 2020 British Academy publication indicated, it would be possible to "recover" and "shape the future" (Few et al., 2020). This crisis account persists today in accounts of the "post-pandemic" world. Yet it has been shadowed and challenged throughout by counteracting accounts of COVID-19 as one of many emergencies within the health and broader ecosphere, geopolitically generated and shaped, with unpredictable and ongoing sequelae; or COVID-19 is seen as a crisis of a different kind, not of health or the economy, but tied to growing and critical levels of inequalities (e.g., Maestripieri, 2021). Is, or was, the COVID-19 pandemic a "crisis"? Does it redefine "crisis" for us or impel us to turn toward a more responsive and dialogic framing of emergency events?

One way to investigate these changing discourses and practices around "crisis" in COVID-19 times is to turn to narrative as an object of study. Narrative was presented from early on in the pandemic as a way to make sense of the individual and larger group meanings of COVID-19; to communicate—especially about science and policy—to varying audiences and to build new knowledge. This chapter focuses on early, dominant COVID-19 narratives within UK government discourse, and counteracting public narrative responses to the pandemic. It also examines counteracting narratives from a less public realm: those emerging from research with people living with HIV—that is, people who are in some ways pandemic experts—about their responses to COVID-19.

The chapter begins by exploring the value of a narrative approach that addresses dominant and counteracting narratives across government,

Corinne Squire, *Dominant and Counteracting Narratives of "Crisis" in COVID Times* In: *Narrative in Crisis.*
Edited by: Martin Dege and Irene Strasser, Oxford University Press. © Oxford University Press 2024.
DOI: 10.1093/oso/9780197751756.003.0004

popular public, and personal COVID-19 stories. It moves on to analyze the value and difficulties of "crisis" versus "emergency" COVID-19 narratives, focusing on dominant UK "slogan" narratives from 2020 and on narratives that counteract them both in the public domain and within research participants' narratives.

Dominant and Counteracting Narratives

One of the ways in which pandemics acquire and accrete meanings is through people, groups, and institutions narrating them into meaning. Mark Davis's and Davina Lohm's recent book *Pandemics, publics, and narrative* (2020) is an excellent introduction to this process. More specifically, Narlikar and Sotilotta (2021) have argued that narratives are key pre-policy elements that politicians have used to shape COVID-19 public attitudes, and Alwan (2021) has analyzed the peer production of long COVID through the gathering and theorizing of testimony. More generally, Carolissen and Kiguwa (2018) and Plummer (2019) argue, what narratives achieve in such a process is a bridging between meanings: subjective meanings become intersubjectively shared, linked to still broader sociopolitical meaning systems, able to gather people together and potentiate action. Supporting these arguments, David Nabarro, one of six Special Envoys to the World Health Organization (WHO) Director-General on COVID-19, narrativized his briefings during the first period of the pandemic—by April 2021, there were 47 such "narratives" (Nabarro, 2021). This WHO approach had the advantage that the briefings could move from level to level of COVID-19 phenomena, hence addressing multiple audiences (Squire et al., 2014).

These features are not, however, the only important elements of narratives for building COVID-19 meanings. Narratives work by building meaning within and across many different kinds of symbol systems, including, in Figure 4.1, a clear and comprehensive "slogan story" of how social and behavioral measures will produce effects constructed across eight words and a meaning-laden design and colorway. Visual narratives have been deployed in COVID-19 education (Jarreau et al., 2021); narratives of COVID-19 loss and grief have been brought together and come together across art, poetry, and other media (Borgstrom & Mallon, 2021).

In these processes, the value of narrative complexity becomes clear (Squire et al., 2014). Such complexity does not, however, just lead to description.

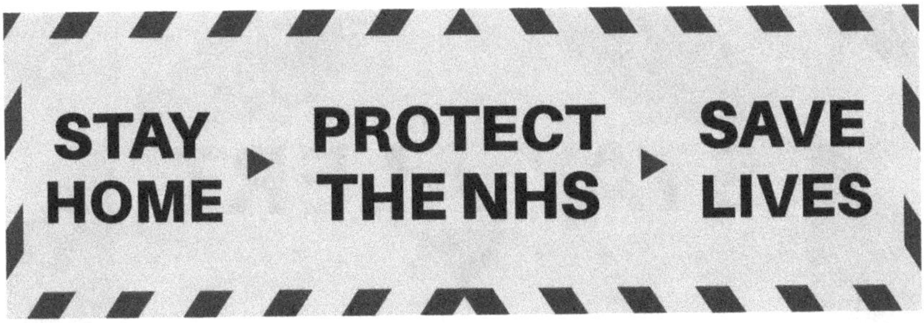

Figure 4.1 UK government COVID-19 slogan, spring 2020.

Narratives try to explain the world, even when, as with the COVID-19 pandemic, many aspects are ambiguous or unknown. Narratives and narrative language itself are therefore causality tales (Squire, 2021). They are complicated, multileveled explanations that express causal relations, including through narrative language itself. They take in political, cultural, historical, social, psychological, and rhetorical as well as biological, chemical, and physical phenomena that determine "human meaning." They are not relativistic in their relation to truth. Some narratives are more truthful, through the breadth and detail of their causal accounts and in their language, and are therefore better and more effective explanations than others.

This chapter focuses on *counteracting* narratives. Counter-narratives and counter-stories (Bamberg & Andrews, 2004; Fine & Harris, 2001; Lueg & Wolff Lundholt, 2021) challenge accepted truths about the world, whether intentionally or not; whether subtly, by implicit transgression (Elliott et al., 2017), or in much more explicit ways (Squire, 2013). Rather than focusing on counter-narratives, their content, and their intent, however, this chapter looks more specifically at *counteracting* narratives. To consider "counteraction" is to foreground the positioning and the processes of narratives: what effects they have (Squire, 2013). Understanding counter-narratives in terms of their effects—as counteracting narratives—means understanding them dialogically. For instance, the Figure 4.2 narrative was unavoidable during summer 2020, in government briefings and in the social and behavioral policies that enacted it. Dylan Patel's (2020) replying tweet used the same visual frame but replaced the words with "BE VAGUE. COVER YOUR BACKS. SHIRK RESPONSIBILITY," and was introduced with the laconic comment, "Fixed it." This counteracting narrative came from a Twitter account with fewer than 1,000 followers. But it was reproduced 2,700 times

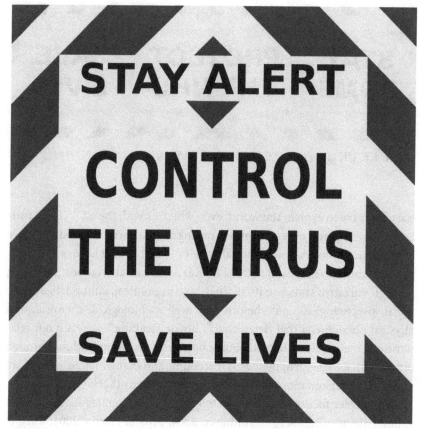

Figure 4.2 UK government.

across social media, and with #StayAlert, it was hash-tagged onto the Figure 4.2 government narrative, giving it an important, community-building currency as a counteracting narrative.

Counteracting narratives may not work directly, as in Patel's parody. They may be more obliquely satirical, as in Sarah Davies's (2020) Twitter image, again responding to Figure 4.2, using its visual framework but replacing the government slogan with the words: "HAVE A BARBEQUE. DO A CONGA. KILL YOUR GRANDMA." They may thus be positioned, As Hage (2015) describes, either as oppositional, like Patel's tweet, or as an "alter" criticism that constitutes a separate reality, a Davies's tweet, does. They may not be effective immediately, or even for a very long time, as

Ahmed (2021) explains in relation to complaint narratives generally. But even counteracting "complaint" narratives still insist on their expression. The furious social media proliferation of alternative slogans along the lines of those above exemplifies such insistence. Counteracting narratives may thus not always be obviously "good" narratives—comprehensive, coherent, or impactful. Yet in the COVID-19 case, acting against hegemonic narratives, we could argue that counteracting narratives are, however imperfect, more inclusive, more qualified—and "better," in the sense of coming closer to the complex truth.

Of course, some counteracting narratives may be effective, but not truthful, as with COVID-19 conspiracy and pseudo-science narratives. Some of the proliferating stories within this field have been partly incorporated into dominant political and policy narratives, but many still operate within counteracting narratives. While it is important to pay serious attention to the truths of, for instance, COVID-19-related economic and geopolitical dispossession, governance failure, personal distress, and underlying politico-economic interests, narratives addressing these factors exclusively remain, though not "post-truth," highly partial truths. The focus of this chapter lies rather with counteracting stories that expand narrative explanation.

Counteracting stories appear in both personal narratives, like those told by individual participants in interview research, and in broader public narratives, such as those appearing in policy documents. These two examples instantiate the differences between the two categories; however, boundaries between the categories are flexible, particularly at a time of large-scale social media personal storytelling, often with extensive reach. And personal narratives of the kind researchers often investigate are themselves rarely only "personal"; they are told to family and friendship networks and often to wider audiences, too. Moreover, stories within different fields intercalate: personal stories are formed by more general, public genres and themselves powerfully shape public stories, so that narratives create heterogeneous, multileveled, but connected "storyworlds" (Herman, 2013; Murray, 2000; Plummer, 2019; Squire, 2013). Consequently, credible narrative research needs to investigate narratives across fields.

In what follows, the chapter analyses examples of counteracting narratives from policy, social media, and an interview study in order to map out how they undo and remake the "crisis" framing of the COVID-19 pandemic.

Interview Study: HIV and COVID-19

The interview study on which the chapter draws analyzes the narratives of 16 participants from a larger study we had conducted in 2019–20 about how people live with HIV and resource constraints. We returned in 2020–2021 to ask how COVID-19 had affected those resource contexts. People with HIV's histories of living with medical uncertainties, fluctuating long-term conditions, loss, denialism, interactions between illness and other inequalities, and the need to act fast and decisively on prevention, testing, treatment, and support—as well as their own awareness of the relevance of their pandemic experience—suggested that they might offer highly salient narratives of this, their second pandemic (Edelman et al., 2020; Gandhi, 2021; Garcia-Iglesias et al., 2021; Hargreaves et al., 2020; HIV Psychosocial Network, 2017). Many people with HIV also live with their own or others' histories of generating counteracting narratives that have impacted HIV prevention, testing, treatment, care, and research, as well as addressing broader injustices around gender, racism, colonialism, and LGBTQ+ rights (Catalan et al., 2020; Epstein, 1998; Mbali, 2013; Powers, 2017; Robins, 2006; Squire, 2013), and that exemplify the continual movements between "personal" and "public" storytelling (Plummer, 2019; Squire, 2013). At the same time, as the COVID-19 pandemic progressed, it became apparent that people who were living with HIV and also with what dominant UK government COVID-19 narratives called "underlying conditions" or "extreme vulnerability," as well as with the multidimensional inequalities shaping the COVID-19 pandemic, might be telling counteracting stories of considerable generality.

In our 2019–20 study, we interviewed people with HIV who already, in many cases, lived with limited health, psychosocial, and other material resources, as well as structural inequalities; it seemed COVID-19 might exacerbate such difficulties (Ambrosiani et al., 2021; Bhaskaran et al., 2020; Brown et al., 2022; Dhairyawan & Chetty, 2020; Petretti et al., 2021; Squire, 2022). We worked with a group roughly equally divided between self-identified gay men, and heterosexual men and women, approximately equally representing majority- and minority-world people, and including mostly people with over five years' experience of living with HIV. We conducted semi-structured telephone interviews lasting between 30 minutes and 2 hours. We analyzed the narratives within the transcripts using a definition of "narratives" as sequences of signs that build meaning through temporal, causal, or spatial sequencing and paying attention to the structural, semantic, and positioning elements of these narratives (Andrews et al., 2013; Squire et al., 2014; Squire, 2021). We also related the narratives in these interviews to those in participants' pre-COVID-19 interviews. Here, we report on two categories of narrative: those told about COVID-19 as a health issue and those told about the COVID-19 future.

Crisis What Crisis?

Illness, Crisis, and Emergency

COVID-19 was classified by the WHO first as a global health emergency, then as a pandemic. Neither term suggests "crisis," a word which in Greek indicates a critical moment in a disease or, more generally, any critical moment where a solution or decision is needed. Rather, a crisis narrative starts before or in the middle of criticality and proceeds through events outside of human control—or, in later uses, events potentially capable of human resolution—to outcome.

Although "crisis" may seem apt for some times within and some aspects of the COVID-19 pandemic, it does not fully explain a situation of general, large-scale, unsettling, but reasoned and widely agreed social response, like that of entering, going through, and emerging from COVID-19 lockdown. Indeed, key early UK academic and policy writing in public health and psychology emerging from the pandemic addressed pandemic preparedness and response and the necessary accompanying community reactions as analyzable and actionable aspects of emergencies, rather than crisis (e.g., Horton, 2020; Jetten et al., 2020). Nor does a crisis narrative provide an account of ongoing COVID-19 uncertainties about how to find, test, trace, isolate, and support effectively the first-identified COVID-19 virus and its variants; treat COVID-19 disease; determine the long-term disease effects; gauge level and length of infection- and vaccine-acquired immunity; discover reasons for global-majority people's comparatively high susceptibilities to serious COVID illness and death in the UK; determine the possible courses of infection and transmission in children; and predict the broader socioeconomic effects of the disease. Uncertainties commonly accompany crisis, especially at the beginning, and here—as is also often reported to be the case—they continue, complicating "crisis" (Crisis and Emergency Risk Communication, 2019). Such continuing uncertainties resonate with the complex interdisciplinary field of counteracting COVID-19 "psychology" narratives just outlined. They cannot simply be assimilated to "crisis"; they turn it into something else.

Crisis, in 19th- and early 20th-century European and North American fiction and nonfiction writing where it is often encountered, is most frequently described as a critical moment in then-fatal illnesses, especially bacterial illnesses, particularly pneumonia. The Canadian physician William Osler described a "fever which usually terminates by crisis" and "self-limited disease" inaccessible to treatment (Osler & McRae, 1921, pp. 78, 101). In Figure 4.3, we see the 1865 pneumonia crisis of Stonewall Jackson, the US Confederate commander, which led to his death. The crisis appears, here as in many representations of the sublime, at the point where pain or sadness, just before the patient reaches a hideous, unrepresentable apogee, can be visually represented as transcendent (Lively, 2013).

Today, by analogy, the term "crisis" is used to describe human and other animal health crises like the Ebola outbreak, severe acute respiratory syndrome (SARS), Middle Eastern respiratory syndrome (MERS), swine flu, bovine spongiform encephalopathy (BSE), and foot and mouth disease, as well as COVID-19; personal crises not associated with illness; climate crisis; a wide range of socioeconomic events like the "refugee crisis" and the "financial crisis"; and even, as this volume's editors mention, disciplinary difficulties—crises in social sciences or psychology. The use of the term "crisis" to describe

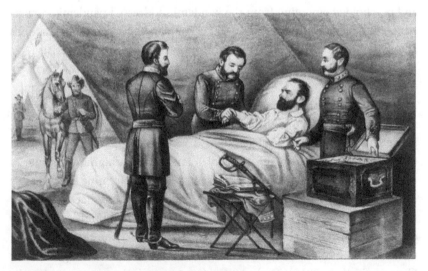

Figure 4.3 Jackson's pneumonia (Lively, 2013).

such eminently solvable biosocial, environmental, political, economic and institutional problems has, not surprisingly, come under criticism (McLean and Rose, 2020; Squire, 1990).

None of these conditions is out of human control in the way pneumonia was (and is still, to some extent, in the case of viral pneumonia). And though COVID-19 pneumonia's early stages and sequelae such as bacterial infections, low oxygen levels, and inflammation can now be treated, future variants and viruses may be more virulent and may escape such treatment. So the viral pneumonia crisis within the COVID-19 pandemic remains to some extent a "crisis" in the first sense of the word. The term "crisis" also applies to other still often medically intractable aspects of COVID-19, like its generation of intense cytokine storm reactions, sepsis, a combination of Kawaski disease and toxic shock syndrome in children, and long COVID.

The other "crises" around COVID-19—for instance, related health and social care system failures, job and productivity losses, steep increases in "mental health" problems, and intensified social inequalities—might better be described, as COVID-19 itself is by the WHO, not as crises but as emergencies: unpredicted happenings that demand immediate attention, about which humans can clearly do something.

Discourse analysts have suggested we study "crisis" not as an inevitability but as discursive construction and social practice (De Rycker, 2018). Some have pointed out the intimate connections of "crises" to current populist politics (Moffitt, 2014). Crisis narratives jibe with political arguments for "disruption" as a means of shifting existing sclerotic economic and administrative structures (Christensen et al., 2018). They can thus be cover stories for other actions—in the United Kingdom, for the government's increased political centralization and healthcare privatization and continued austerity policies. Similarly, they may allow organizations to address preexisting problems under their rubric. As Deloitte put it in 2017, foreshadowing its rapid and profitable UK move into COVID-19 consultancy and testing, "resilient leaders use (crisis) as an opportunity to fix things that aren't working, go from defense to offense—and emerge in a way that ultimately makes the organization stronger" (Deloitte, 2017, p. 3).

Forced migrants and forced migration scholars have often refused the term "crisis" due to its naturalizing qualities, which suggest that nothing can be done about a situation (Krzyzanowsi et al., 2018). To some extent, an environmental emergency may already be beyond human control. However, the term "crisis" can overgeneralize those aspects of uncontrollability, as environmental campaigners like Greta Thunberg recognize when they concentrate on narratives of successful past, present, and future interventions.

Pandemics and other serious illness outbreaks are, currently, largely recoverable situations, given widely understood, developed, and practiced public health principles—more like emergencies than crises. The term "crisis" is not wrong in these situations, but it seems useful to think about how exactly it is working.

A pandemic can then also be narrated as an emergency: not a "crisis" singularity that can be solved or resolved, but an ongoing event or set of events, to some extent unpredicted, that require continuing and multiple focuses of attention. This description comes close, in its complexity and contestation, to the counteracting narratives of COVID-19 "psychology" explored above.

"Stay Home": Dominant Governmental and Counteracting Popular and Personal Narratives of COVID-Era Health

In the United Kingdom, the dominant discourse in government, policy, and media around COVID-19—until the arrival of effective vaccines in early to mid-2021—was indeed that of crisis expressed in the "slogan" narratives shown in Figures 4.1 and 4.2. These two narratives and the public and personal narratives that arose to counteract them demonstrate the contradictions and undoings of COVID's "crisis" framing.

The first slogan narrative (Figure 4.1) appeared in the context of high and rising COVID-19 infections, hospitalizations, and deaths, and the impending overwhelming of the National Health Service (NHS). It moved to the resolution of that "crisis" by the partial mitigating implementation of public health principles—a medium-strength lockdown, physical distancing, and sanitation, to avoid aerosol and fomite transmission, alongside the maintenance of education, labor, and consumer activities at lowered levels. This was the "Stay Home, Save the NHS, Save Lives" story, a foreshadowing narrative (Brockmeier, 2015) that both ordered and projected the immediate future, articulated first in March 2020.

Successful slogan narratives are agreed upon by those working with them in, for example public health, fundraising, and advertising, to have common features: simplicity, conciseness, clarity, consistency, specificity, empowerment, and action orientation (Lee & Spanier, 2020; Oerther & Watson, 2020). These features can interact well with the

straightforwardness and urgency of a crisis situation. But the simple se-
quence of "Stay Home, Protect the NHS, Save Lives" obfuscated some necessarily complex arguments—in the process, casting doubt on dominant
narratives' "crisis" framing of COVID-19.

For instance, the simplicity of "Stay Home" required qualification—"Stay
Home" unless you have to go to work, are unsafe at home, are a special-
category child who can attend school, for daily exercise, for basic shop-
ping, or to provide essential care—which might more effectively have been
addressed by attentive, detailed explication within an "emergency" narrative. A failure of public trust (Enria et al., 2021), expressed in counteracting
stories of anger and disappointment that powerful people did not enact the
dominant narrative, followed, most notably, government advisor Dominic
Cummings's failure to "stay home"—his travel between London, Durham,
and Barnard Castle and his stay in Durham, all of which he justified by, precisely, care responsibilities. This counteracting psychopolitical "low trust"
narrative indicated the problems of relying on a "crisis" narrative that was
never as universal as it declared, and was followed by longlasting expressions
of declines in public trust (Edelman et al., 2020).

In addition, it seemed that, some weeks before the government's "Stay
Home, Protect the NHS, Save Lives" narrative, people were telling and
living out this narrative already, counteracting what they viewed as government complacency. They decided to stay home, take children out of school,
leave universities, absent themselves from transport and retail spaces, and
close offices (BBC, 2020; Jetten et al., 2020). "Stay Home, Protect the NHS,
Save Lives" thus relied heavily for its success on people's already-formulated
narratives of action and empowerment. This popular enacted narrative was
indeed timed around right. National lockdown at this time, as happened
in Germany, would have avoided the first wave of exponential community
transmission in the United Kingdom.

Third, "Stay Home, Protect the NHS, Save Lives" lacked clarity, despite its
brevity; it was three stories in one. For the government, it ran linearly from
staying home to reduce infections, even if ill, to reducing NHS pressure, to
allowing hospitals to treat the most life-threatening COVID-19 infections
and not appear, as in Italy, as failed spaces of abjection and death. For many
public audiences, though, the story disaggregated into two counteracting
narratives: (1) "Stay home, Protect the NHS" a self-contained, COVID-19-
independent narrative, commensurate with the NHS's highly valued social
protection function in the United Kingdom; and (2) "Stay Home, Save Lives"

a story of avoiding infection and thereby serious illness and death, rather than simply reducing infection so the NHS could cope with serious illness.

We may gain an even stronger sense of counteracting narratives of "crisis" framings of COVID-19 by considering the extended and complex personal narratives that people tell to friends, family, themselves—and to researchers—about their COVID-19-era thoughts, feelings, and actions.

When narrating their understandings of COVID-19 as a health issue, all 16 participants in the "living with HIV and COVID-19" study recounted having good COVID-19 knowledge and reducing risk as much as possible, in accordance with WHO and independent, nongovernmental UK public health advice. These narratives thus counteracted the "Stay Home" story's ambiguity about reducing infection risk, without referencing it, through "alter" public health accounts of taking people's own, independently verified precautionary measures.

Anabella, for example, narrated her care during the first lockdown to go out as rarely as possible, always masked, avoid areas where aerosolized transmission might happen, clean public spaces in her housing, and gather information from all possible sources—even though government narratives did not advise masking against aerosol transmission, but only emphasized droplet transmission and were vague about fomite transmission, This narrative work was also shared, done with and to protect Anabella's friends.

ANABELLA: I am on A (floor), and there are people on B (floor). /mhm/ So, we use the same door. We have the communal landing /yeah/ so we use the same door, and there are more people on B, I think they are more than three anyway /I see/ so yeah, they keep going in and out, unlike me, I'm in all the time, so when they (), their girlfriends, when they step into the communal landing, then they sneeze, then they cough /right/ they don't know about the scary part of it.

INTERVIEWER: Yeah, sure. Are you uh, are you taking you know, precautions hygiene-wise, is that for you're—?

P4F3: Yes, actually, I'm actually very good at that /mhm/ I don't hold the door handles with my hands. Um, when I get time, I sanitise the, you know, I use the wipes /yeah/ to wipe them and every time I go out, I get a tissue and then you know, put the tissue on my face and then open the door, you know /of course/ yeah, that's what I try, by all means. . . . I remember one of the rules said people should not go to the parks and in my mind I'm saying I should not go to the park because I say we should be safe, you know /yeah/ we should not travel unnecessarily /yes/ we should stay safe, so I haven't been to the park so far /ah yeah/ just to go and get the sunshine /yes/. . . . I know a lot of people have actually died and um, yeah, it's like I'm trying to be extra careful not to be the next one, you know /of course/ even not to try and be get the virus and take it to the next (support group) session you know.

"Stay Alert": Dominant Government and Counteracting Popular and Personal Narratives

The UK government's second 2020 slogan narrative appeared as cases—and deaths—fell in summer and amid a declared "new crisis" or, in some accounts, "pandemic" of lockdown-associated recession, poverty, and mental distress; increased social inequalities; and non-COVID-19-related illnesses and deaths. The government narrated this double crisis as resolvable via a "learning to live with the virus" process, normalizing return to work, education, consumption, and continuing disease risk alongside some continuing public health mitigation. The slogan narrative expressing this policy, "Stay Alert, Control the Virus, Save Lives," seen in Figure 4.2, was now color-coded benignly, "green for go" replacing "red for stop."

This move was a departure from the WHO and most other public health guidelines still emphasizing pandemic suppression, in favor of a perhaps deliberately vague "management" of the virus. It broke a number of public health and other communication rules. It was not consistent with the prior message; it was concise and simple but not clear; and its relations to affect, except for the unambiguous good of saving lives and action—but how, exactly, to stay alert, control a virus, save lives?—were murky. Within a crisis narrative, that imprecision allowed space for many interpretations, particularly at a time of medical uncertainty, socioeconomic precarity and loss, and psychological distress. "Stay alert" called up prior alerts about enemies within and without, around war and terrorism (Welshman, 2020). "Control the virus" required personal action over an invisible, submicroscopic entity. This "crisis" slogan narrative thus undid itself with its imprecision.

Counteracting narratives responded immediately to this second slogan narrative. As in Figure 4.3, oppositional parodic and satirical rewritings erupted, pointing up the slogan's communicative failures, political blame-shifting, and eugenicist undertones. Lived counteracting narratives of an alter-reality—of continuing to stay home, save the NHS, and save lives—also appeared in, for instance, opinion polls showing no change from pre-lockdown in people thinking that health outweighed the economy as a policy priority (Reicher, 2021; Skinner & Pedley, 2020), and in widespread parental, professional, local authority, and union resistance to, for instance, reopening schools. The effectiveness of these counteracting narratives was perhaps indicated in government responses that frequently hit back at critically cautious narrators as psychopathologically fearful of risk.

The counteracting "future" narratives that four participants generated in the HIV and COVID-19 study around lockdown-lifting stuck with the prior but now-tangential "Stay Home, Save Lives" narrative direction, which by now constituted a kind of alter-reality, again without referencing the dominant political story. These narratives were also shared in virtual support groups and informal networks and supported continuing caution. These participants were not using public transport; they continued remote working if they had non-frontline work; they did not "eat out to help out." Anabella told this story of her planned understanding and actions up until the end of 2020—again, a story shared and developed with her friendship networks.

ANABELLA: Yes, yes, I've actually thought about it (the post-lockdown future). To me, I feel still, like today I'm carrying one now, I (will) still put on my mask, I still keep the social distance, because um when they lift the lockdown, it will not mean that the virus is expired because that it has come to an end, no. They, which means, the virus will still be there so it's up to me really to still be, you know, to uh to still take precautions like um, do exactly like the way I'm doing now and until it is properly confirmed by the end of the year or the next year that no more cases have been reported then maybe I can try and get closer to people and give them a hug {laughs}

More generally, 12 participants told counteracting stories about a future "opening up" that would offer a "new normal," sometimes explicitly contrasted with, although not criticizing, the return to "normal" postulated in government narratives. Three of these stories also predicted economic "belt-tightening." Joe Blogs, like most, postulated a postponed and different sociality, a future story he also developed dialogically on social media.

JOE BLOGS: What will things be like? Will there be a normal? I do wonder if afterwards, are there gonna be, is it gonna cause to be some changes in those kinda (things)/yeah/ you know and which, in some ways will be a benefit and then in other ways, wou-, would you know would, it might have a downside as well and then, I don't know, I think it's gonna take time, I think it's gonna take time and /mhm/ it'll be interesting what the government are doing and just in, being able to go to the cinema again or go to the theatre, um, you know to do all the things /yeah, yes/ that I love doing you know, which have just, which have just totally stopped you know completely. And it's, you think that it's just sitting in the cinema, you know, how close you get to the person in the next seat /sure/ you know, it's pretty close {chuckles} /yes/ you know, it's gonna be interesting to see how, how I would feel sitting you know in the cinema that close to people you know, after this, um and when that would seem normal again, /mhm/ I think that will take time. /yeah/

Finally, Joseph articulated a time-unlimited counteracting narrative. The ongoing "new normal" uncertainties he was contemplating were of a general kind and involved ongoing preparedness for possible future pandemics—a level of foresight that still, towards the end of 2023, lies outside of government narratives. At the same time, Joseph was planning a personal reconnection with the world—though not the labor and consumption re-engagement urged by the government. And he was developing this counteracting narrative with his support group, extending its effectiveness to the collectivities around him.

JOSEPH: I had a meeting a few month ago . . . (we) said you know "nothing is going to be okay"/uhuh/and this was way before this (pandemic . . . we are never going to be totally okay/uhuh/there is always going to be stuff and I think I've always been sort of reflecting on that/right/uhuh/. . . . And I'm actually thinking of opening an online profile, and I think it (the pandemic) has had that effect where it makes me think, "Oh why don't I just get over myself and get on with it" (Laughs), because you know life is short and it could be nice, I think I've overcome the sort of fear out of it.

In these counteracting narratives, rather than reiterating or opposing the government's new "crisis" framing, participants are creating alter narratives (Hage, 2015). They narrate futures extended and qualified long and far

64 CORINNE SQUIRE

beyond "crisis." These stories picture a continuing state of emergency within which participants narrate their and their social networks' own imagined material, social, and personal futures into possible action.

Conclusion

This chapter has argued for the value of considering counteracting (Squire, 2013) rather than simply counter-narratives of COVID-19 "psychology" and "crisis" framings. It has analyzed counteracting narratives as complex and truth-pursuing through their positioning, processes, and effects—as constituted by what they do, rather than only by what they say. While narratives' counteracting impacts are difficult to register fully within social research, the chapter suggests that some partial mapping of both "public" and "personal" narratives' counteracting effects is possible. The chapter also indicates that analyzing counteracting narratives of the COVID-19 crisis across the fields of social media, policy, and personal storytelling shows processes of marked similarities across these "storyworlds," which supports the value of analytic approaches spanning these narrative fields.

In analyzing counteracting narratives, the chapter has identified "alter" more than "oppositional" constructions of COVID-19's "crisis" framing. These counteracting narratives, rather than directly combatting dominant narratives, set them aside to generate alternative representational worlds. Such preponderance of "alter" counteracting narratives supports Hage's (2015) emphasis on alter-criticisms as what he suggests are neglected forms of political engagement.

The chapter has drawn on the counteracting narratives of COVID-19 told by people with HIV. People with HIV live with particular histories of biomedicine, illness, socioeconomic disadvantage, intersectionalities, stigma, and pandemic which render their COVID-19 stories especially relevant (Garcia-Iglesias et al., 2021). Yet, in their counteracting narrations of COVID-19, they seem to express some commonalities with those who are now living with other long-term conditions and disabilities alongside COVID-19—for instance, those living with myalgic encephalomyelitis (ME) or chronic fatigue syndrome (CFS) (Gallagher & Voela, 2021)—as well as with those living with the multidimensional inequalities that have exacerbated COVID-19's effects. People with HIV thus speak at an intersection of histories of pandemic and systems of structural disadvantage, which makes them important narrators within the COVID-19 pandemic.

The chapter has shown how counteracting narratives, both "public" and "personal," can work against the government's dominant, crisis-framed narratives of COVID-19. Crisis narratives are often straightforward, concise, and mobilizing. But they can also, as this chapter has argued, be too simplifying and totalizing to address adequately complex public health issues like the COVID-19 pandemic. In such circumstances, the alternative "emergency" narratives described here can serve as counteracting stories that criticize and complicate and, in the process, produce fuller narrative truths, in representations and in other forms of actions.

"Crisis" may still have a place in how we understand this pandemic. We might, for instance, draw on Gramsci's (1971; Hall & Massey, 2010) account of crisis as, first of all, process, with its own history; as organic; and as characterized by morbid symptoms. The COVID-19 pandemic event is indeed part of a much longer process of human environmental and colonial exploitation through which both the asset-stripped planet and the disempowered majority world have lost the "right to breathe" as surely as do those with COVID-19 who are deprived of oxygen, adequate hospital care, or lung function (Mbembe, 2020). Within the long-running processes of this global neoliberal environmental and sociopolitical "crisis," many reactions to COVID-19, especially far-right and post-truth counteracting narratives (Babic, 2020), could be said to be "morbid symptoms." The counteracting narratives described in this chapter are, however, more like indices of the long-running crisis's organicity as they powerfully articulate "alter" realities tangential to dominant orders of governance and representation. It is important to recognize that progressive counteracting narratives, oriented toward social justice and care, like the ones described here in both personal and public fields, are today, mainly, only effective in this tangential way, outside of the dominant narratives of governmentality. The counteracting alter-narratives described above thus index a crisis much larger than the COVID-19 event whose "crisis" status they disassemble.

Acknowledgments

Thanks to Jamilson Bernardo De Lemos, Tina Franklin, Ceasar Kalema, Vanessa Kellerman, Abu Talha Al-Hussain and Treasure Zulu, in the UK, and to Floretta Boonzaier, Nondumiso Hlwele, Ivan Katsere, Sanny Mulubale, Simone Peters, and Adriana Prates, working on the sister projects in South Africa, Zambia, and Brazil.

References

Ahmed, S. (2021). *Complaint!* Duke University Press.

Alwan, N. (2021). The road to addressing long COVID. *Science, 373*(6554), 491–493.

Ambrosioni, J., Blanco, L., Reyes-Urueña, J., Davies, M-A., Sued, O., Marcos, M., Martínez, E., Bertagnolio, S., Alcamí, J., & Miro, J. (2021). Overview of SARS-CoV-2 infection in adults living with HIV. *Lancet, 8*(5), E294–E305.

Andrews, M., Squire, C., & Tamboukou, M. (2013). *Doing Narrative Research.* London: Sage.

Babic, M. (2020). Let's talk about the interregnum. *International Affairs, 96*(3), 767–786.

Bamberg, M., & Andrews, M. (2004). *Considering counter-narratives.* Benjamins.

BBC. (2020, March 16). Coronavirus: London tube passenger numbers fall during outbreak. https://www.bbc.co.uk/news/uk-england-london-51910740

Bhaskaran, K., Rentsch, C., MacKenna, B., Schulze, A., Mehrkar, A., Bates, C., et al. (2020). HIV infection and COVID-19 death. *Lancet, 8*(1), E24–E32.

Borgstrom, E., & Mallon, S. (2021). *Milton Keynes: The Open University.*

Brockmeier, J. (2015). *Beyond the archive.* Oxford University Press.

Brown, A., Croxford, S., Nash, S., Khawam, J., Kirwan, P., Kall, M., et al. (2022, January). COVID-19 mortality among people with diagnosed HIV compared to those without during the first wave of the COVID-19 pandemic in England, *HIV Medicine, 23*, 90–102.

Carolissen, R., & Kiguwa, P. (2018). Narrative explorations of the micro-politics of students' citizenship, belonging and alienation at South African universities. *South African Journal of Higher Education, 32*(3), 1–111.

Catalan, J., Hedge, B., & Ridge, D. (2020). *HIV in the UK: Voices from the epidemic.* Routledge.

Christensen, C., McDonald, R., Altman, E., & Palmer, J. (2018, June 16). Disruptive innovation. *Journal of Management Studies.* https://onlinelibrary.wiley.com/doi/full/10.1111/joms.12349

Crisis and Emergency Risk Communication. (2019). Psychology of a crisis. Centers for Disease Control. https://emergency.cdc.gov/cerc/ppt/CERC_Psychology_of_a_Crisis.pdf

Davies, S. (2020, May 11). Sarah Davies . . . Socialist @sarah_davies67. "HAVE A BARBEQUE. DO A CONGA. KILL YOUR GRANDMA'. 1.15 PM Tweet. https://twitter.com/sarah_davies67/status/1259819381401550855

Davis, M., & Lohm, D. (2020). *Pandemics, publics, and narrative.* Oxford University Press.

Deloitte. (2017). The next wave. https://www2.deloitte.com/content/dam/Deloitte/us/Documents/risk/us-risk-emerging-stronger-from-crisis.pdf

De Rycker, A. (2018, January). The crisis-discourse dialectic. *Journal of Services and Management, 9*, 73–83.

Dhairyawan, R., & Chetty, D. (2020, April 15). COVID-19, racism, and health outcomes. *Discover Society.* https://archive.discoversociety.org/2020/04/15/covid-19-racism-and-health-outcomes/

Edelman, J., Aoun-Barakat, L., Villanueva, M., & Friedland, G. (2020). Confronting another pandemic. *AIDS and Behavior, 24*, 1977–1979.

Elliott, H., O'Connell, R., & Squire, C. (2017). Narratives of normativity and permissible
transgression. *FQS,18*, 1. https://www.qualitative-research.net/index.php/fqs/article/
view/2775

Enria, L., Waterlow, N., Rogers, N., Brindle, H., Lal, S., Eggo, R. M., Lees, S., & Roberts, C.
(2021). Trust and transparency in times of crisis. London School of Hygiene & Tropical
Medicine, London, United Kingdom. https://doi.org/10.17037/DATA.00002015

Epstein, S. (1998). *Impure science.* University of California Press.

Few, R., Chhotray, V., Tebboth, M., Forster, J., White, C., Teresa Armijos, T., & Shelton, C.
(2020). COVID-19 crisis: Lessons for recovery. British Academy. https://www.thebri
tishacademy.ac.uk/publications/covid-19-crisis-lessons-recovery/

Fine, M., & Harris, A. (2001). *Under the covers: Theorising the politics of counter stories.*
Lawrence and Wishart.

Gallagher, S., & Voela, A. (2021). In D. Ellis and A. Voela (Eds.), *After lockdown: Opening
up.* Palgrave Macmillan.

Gandhi, M. (2021, April 26). Four ways HIV activists have saved lives during COVID.
Poz, April 26. https://www.poz.com/article/four-ways-hiv-activists-saved-lives-covid.

Garcia-Iglesias, J., Nagington, M., & Aggleton, P. (2021). Viral times, viral memories, viral
questions. *Culture, Health and Sexuality, 23*(11),1465–1469.

Gramsci, A. (1971). *Selections from the prison notebooks.* International Publishers.

Hage, G. (2015). *Alter-politics.* Manchester University Press.

Hall, S., & Massey, D. (2010). Interpreting the crisis. *Soundings, 44*, 57–71.

Hargreaves, J., Davey. C.; Group for lessons from pandemic HIV prevention for the
COVID-19 response (2020, May). Three lessons for the COVID-19 response from
pandemic HIV. *Lancet HIV, 7*(5), e309–e311.

Herman, D. (2013). Approaches to narrative worldmaking. In M. Andrews, C. Squire, and
M. Tamboukou (Eds.), *Doing narrative research* (pp. 176–196). London: Sage.

HIV Psychosocial Network. (2017). Ten years after: An 'austerity audit'of services and
living conditions for people living with HIV in the UK, a decade after the financial
crisis. https://hivpsychosocialnetworkuk.files.wordpress.com/2018/11/10-years-after-
final.pdf. Accessed 05.10.23.

Horton, R. (2020). *The COVID-19 catastrophe.* Polity.

Jarreau, P., Su, L., Chiang, E., Bennett, S., Zhang, J., Ferguson, M., & Algarra, D. (2021,
August 18). Visual narratives about COVID-19 improve message accessibility, self-
efficacy, and health precautions. *Frontiers in Communication.* https://www.frontiersin.
org/articles/10.3389/fcomm.2021.712658/full

Jetten, J., Reicher, S., Haslam, A., & Cruwys, T. (2020). *Together apart.* Sage.

Krzyzanowski, M., Triandafyllidou, A., & Wodak, R. (2018, February 28). The
mediatisation and the politicisation of the "refugee crisis" in Europe. *Journal of
Immigrant and Refugee Studies, 16*(1–14). https://www.tandfonline.com/doi/full/
10.1080/15562948.2017.1353189

Lee, J., & Spanier, G. (2020, May 11). "Single-minded and unavoidable": How the government honed "Stay home" message. https://www.campaignlive.co.uk/article/single-min
ded-unavoidable-government-honed-stay-home-message/1682448

Lively, M. (2013, May 13). "The most fatal of all acute diseases": Pneumonia and the death
of Stonewall Jackson. *Civil War Monitor.* https://www.civilwarmonitor.com/blog/the-
most-fatal-of-all-acute-diseases-pneumonia-and-the-death-of-stonewall-jackson

Lueg, K., & Wolff Lundholt, M. (2021). *Routledge handbook of counter-narratives*. Routledge.

Maetripieri, L. (2021, May 26). The COVID-19 pandemics. *Frontiers in Sociology*. https://www.frontiersin.org/articles/10.3389/fsoc.2021.642662/full

Mbali, M. (2013). *South African AIDS activism and global health politics*. Palgrave

Mbembe, A. (2020) The universal right to breathe. *Critical Inquiry, 47*. https://www.journals.uchicago.edu/doi/full/10.1086/711437. Accessed 05.10.23.

McLean, S., & Rose, N. (2020). Crisis, what crisis? Addiction neuroscience and the challenges of translation. *Wellcome Open Research, 5*(215), 1–20. https://doi.org/10.12688/wellcomeopenres.16265.1

Moffitt, B. (2014, May 29). How to perform crisis. *Government and Opposition* 50(2). https://www.cambridge.org/core/journals/government-and-opposition/article/how-to-perform-crisis-a-model-for-understanding-the-key-role-of-crisis-in-contemporary-populism/3A522C020FF774CFA5D0C91CD10A98F1

Murray, M. (2000). Levels of narrative analysis in health psychology. *Journal of Health Psychology, 5*(3), 337–347.

Nabarro, D. (2021). COVID 19 narratives by Dr. David Nabarro. 4SD. https://www.4sd.info/covid-19-narratives/)

Narlikar, A., & Sottilotta, C. E. (2021). Pandemic narratives and policy responses. *Journal of European Public Policy, 28*(8), 1238–1257.

Oerther, D., & Watson, R. (2020, August 10). Risk communication is important for environmental engineering during COVID 19. *Journal of Environmental Engineering, 146*, 10. https://ascelibrary.org/doi/full/10.1061/%28ASCE%29EE.1943-7870.0001796. Accessed 05.10.23.

Osler, W., & McRae, T. (1921). *The principles and practice of medicine*. Appleton.

Patel, D. (2020). Tweet. https://twitter.com/dylan_patel. Dylan / ЄℓＱ⁻ℓ@dylan_patel. (2020, May 10). Fixed it. This government is doing the bare minimum it can get away with so that at the inevitable public enquiry, they can shrug and say 'we did run a comms campaign, not our fault if nobody followed the advice'. StayAlert. BE VAGUE. COVER OUR BACKS. SHIRK RESPONSIBILITY. 8:19 AM Tweet. https://twitter.com/dylan_patel/status/1259382422048854016

Petretti, S., O'Hanlon, C., Brough, G., Bruton, J., Squire, C., & Tariq, S. (2021). "For me, it is my second pandemic": Experiences of people living with HIV accessing support from Positively UK during COVID 19. BHIVA annual conference. https://www.bhiva.org/file/60c0b0f70a526/P130.pdf

Plummer, K. (2019). *Narrative power*. Sage.

Powers, T. (2017). *Sustaining life*. University of Pennsylvania Press.

Reicher, S. (2021, January 7). Pandemic fatigue? *The BMJ Opinion*. blogs.bmj.com/bmj/2021/01/07/pandemic-fatigue-how-adherence-to-covid-19-regulations-has-been-misrepresented-and-why-it-matters/

Robins, S. (2006). *From revolution to rights in South Africa*. James Currey.

Skinner, G., & Pedley, K. (2020, May 12). Majority of Britons continue to think the government should prioritise health over economy in COVID-19 response. Ipsos Mori. https://www.ipsos.com/ipsos-mori/en-uk/majority-britons-continue-think-government-should-prioritise-health-over-economy-covid-19-response

Squire, C. (1990). Crisis what crisis? In I. Parker & J. Shotter (Eds.), *Deconstructing social psychology*. Routledge.

Squire, C. (2013). *Living with HIV and ARV*. Palgrave.

Squire, C. (Ed.). (2021). *Stories changing lives*. Oxford University Press.

Squire, C. (Forthcoming). Narrating resistant citizenships through two pandemics.

Squire, C., Davis, M., Esin, C., Harrison, B., Hyden, L.-C., & Hyden, M. (2014). *What is narrative research?* Bloomsbury.

Welshman, R. (2020, May 13). Dangerous and subversive: The government's new "Stay Alert" COVID-19 messaging. *Byline Times*. https://bylinetimes.com/2020/05/12/dangerous-and-subversive-the-uk-governments-new-stay-alert-covid-19-messaging/

5

The Pandemic as a Crossroads

Problematizing the Narrative of War

Hanna Meretoja

Military metaphors dominate public imagination concerning serious illnesses. We are all familiar with references to "war on cancer" and someone "losing their battle to serious illness." Hence, it was hardly surprising that when the COVID-19 pandemic erupted in early 2020, it was quickly framed in terms of a narrative of war. Although there has been, by now, much criticism of this narrative that has dominated public discourse on the pandemic, there is still a need for a more acute understanding of the different aspects that make it problematic.[1] Our thinking is inevitably metaphorical and mediated by cultural narratives, so I am not suggesting that we could try to avoid all metaphors and narratives in discussing the pandemic, but it is important to be aware of which narratives we use and to evaluate whether they do more good or harm. In this chapter, I provide grounds for understanding the harmfulness of the war narrative by analyzing problems in the way it ascribes agency to the coronavirus, healthcare professionals, patients, and the public as a whole. In the end, I propose an alternative narrative framework that revolves around the idea of humanity at a historical crossroads. This chapter thereby not only contributes to the study of the dangers of narratives (see Fernandes, 2017; Mäkelä & Meretoja, 2022; Meretoja, 2018) but also questions the dominant view of narratives as retrospective accounts of events and experiences.

---

[1] The first analyses of the problems in the war narrative were published in spring 2020 (see Fairbanks, 2020; Meretoja, 2020, on which I draw and expand in this chapter; Wilkinson, 2020), and Spanish scholars initiated #ReframeCovid, which invited people to suggest alternatives to the military metaphors in an open-source document.

Hanna Meretoja, *The Pandemic as a Crossroads* In: *Narrative in Crisis*. Edited by: Martin Dege and Irene Strasser, Oxford University Press. © Oxford University Press 2024. DOI: 10.1093/oso/9780197751756.003.0005

The Narrative of War

As soon as the gravity of the situation became clear, the narrative of war emerged as the dominant way of framing the pandemic through a series of grandiose gestures by world leaders. President Donald Trump (2020a, 2020b) branded himself as a "wartime president" and called the pandemic "the worst attack" ever on the United States." Prime Minister Boris Johnson (2020a) took on a Churchillian pose by declaring: "We must act like any wartime government." Later, he described the virus as an "alien invader," confident that the United Kingdom would repel it as it has seen off all invaders "for the last thousand years" (Johnson, 2020b). President Emmanuel Macron (2020) asserted multiple times in his televised speech: "We are at war." President Joe Biden (2021) is now using the rhetoric of war just as passionately as his predecessor: during his first days in office, he pledged a "full-scale wartime effort" to combat the virus. All these leaders launched a war against an "invisible enemy." The media and health organizations also adopted the military vocabulary of doctors fighting on the "frontline" and of "an army of volunteers" helping the British National Health Service in the joint war effort (NHS, 2020).

Leaders have political reasons to use the language of war. Historically, wartime leaders have been popular, a joint enemy creates national unity, and the comparison to a war conveys the gravity of the situation. The trope of war is also a way of justifying emergency legislation and suspension of certain civil liberties. Some commentators have suggested that war can be an empowering metaphor.[2] Its appeal is understandable because it turns us from passive victims to courageous soldiers in a fight against a common enemy, but it is nevertheless a deeply problematic narrative. By ascribing agency to "us," the narrative of battle functions as a means of creating an illusion of control. In this chapter, I analyze why such an illusion of control is problematic—not only because it gives a false sense of security but also because, overall, instead of warmongering, a more productive response to the pandemic as a global

---

[2] Semino (2021) discusses the empowering potential of the war metaphor and suggests that it may have been "appropriate at the beginning of the pandemic, to convey the dangers posed by the virus, justify the need for radical changes in lifestyle, and generate a sense of collective responsibility and sacrifice for a common purpose," but she also acknowledges that it has dangers and limitations, such as creating "excessive anxiety, potentially legitimizing authoritarian governmental measures." On the retraumatizing potential of the language of war for those who have experienced an actual war, see Martínez García (2021) and Banjeglav and Moll (2021).

crisis would be one that acknowledges the limits of our agency and the need to learn humility and respect for non-human nature.

Others have observed that war functions as a key *metaphor* when the pandemic is framed as war.[3] In what sense does war also function as a *narrative* in this context? I suggest that war functions as a *narrative model of sense-making* that guides the way we think about the pandemic. In my earlier research, I have proposed conceptualizing narrative as an *interpretative activity of cultural sense-making,* in which experiences are presented to someone from a certain *perspective* as part of a *meaningful, connected account,* which is relevant for our understanding of *human possibilities* (Meretoja, 2018, p. 48). Narratives can expand or diminish our "sense of the possible" (pp. 90–97), and this is crucial for evaluating what different narratives do to us. The approach that I, together with others, have called *narrative hermeneutics* (see Brockmeier, 2015; Brockmeier & Meretoja, 2014; Freeman, 2015; Meretoja, 2014, 2018) emphasizes that narrative is precisely a culturally mediated *interpretative activity.* As the phenomenologist Edmund Husserl (2006, p. 250) made clear, "something as something" (*etwas als etwas*), the basic structure of interpretation, characterizes even simple sense perception.[4] Narratives make sense of the narrated events, experiences, or phenomena by interpreting them from certain perspectives that foreground what particular individuals experience in particular situations to which they respond. Narratives are entangled with power, such as questions of who gets to decide whose experiences are narrated and how. Narratives are never ethically neutral (Ricoeur, 1992, p. 140). Crucial to how a narrative is framed is the act of ascribing agency—laying out who the central agents are and who did what. If a narrative activates a certain narrative model of sense-making, it activates our *narrative assumptions* on what kinds of actors are involved, how the action is likely to unfold, what possible scenarios it may follow, and so on.[5]

Most often the narrative of war is an *implicit* narrative, one that functions as a model of sense-making, underlying specific narratives but rarely told anywhere in a fully fleshed out textual form.[6] It guides us to cast certain actors in certain roles and creates narrative assumptions such as that there is a war between "us" and "them," us and the enemy. It also creates the expectation

---

[3] See, e.g., Semino, 2021, and the #ReframeCovid initiative.

[4] For example, we see a tree *as* a tree, whereby the concept of a tree organizes the sense perception. On "something *as* something" as primordial to "our world orientation," see Gadamer, 1984, p. 58.

[5] On narrative assumptions, see Meretoja, 2021, 38–39.

[6] I theorize the distinction between implicit and explicit narratives in Meretoja (2021, 2023a).

of a temporal development: from a declaration of war to drawing up a war strategy and tactics, fighting key battles, developing new weapons, mourning sacrifices that are necessary in any war—a narrative arch extending all the way to an ending that is either a victory or a defeat. The narrative of war casts the key actors in the role of soldiers. In the pandemic war narrative, there are four groups of actors that play the role of soldier: first, the coronavirus; second, healthcare workers; third, patients; and fourth, the public as a whole. Each of these ascriptions of agency is highly problematic.

The Virus as an Enemy Combatant

First, the narrative of war ascribes agency to the coronavirus. It is indeed a central agent in the pandemic, but the problem is that the narrative of war anthropomorphizes the virus. It casts the virus in the role of an enemy, one that is a human-like other. The virus is said to have plans and strategies; it is described as clever in its ability to mutate and in its efforts to resist our strategies to defeat it.

A good example of the public discourse that casts the virus in the role of an enemy combatant is an article in the *New York Magazine*, in March 2020: "How the coronavirus could take over your body (before you ever feel it)" by Jeff Wise (2020). It narrates in detail how the virus intrudes the body and begins its attack on the first lung cell: "A billion years of evolution have equipped it to resist attackers. But it also has a vulnerability—a backdoor." As soon as the combatant "is in," it begins to "hijack" lung cells and replicate its genetic material: "All up and down your lungs, throat, and mouth, the scene is repeated over and over as cell after cell is penetrated and hijacked." Quickly, a full-fledged war is storming through the body: "Within your body, a microscopic Battle of the Somme is raging with your immune system leveling its Big Berthas on both the enemy trenches and its own troops." It is a morality tale in which the clever virus combatant takes over the body of an arrogant young man and the transmission chain leads back to "the wife of a cryptocurrency speculator."

In biology and medicine, military metaphors have a long history (see, e.g., Bleakley, 2017). The human immune system is commonly thought of in terms of a constant war against harmful intruders. Scientists say that the genetic program of pathogens "orders" them to "hijack" and eventually kill the host cells in order to ensure their own chances to reproduce and invade new organisms. We are so used to such a manner of speech that often we do not even notice the anthropomorphization and the military vocabulary. The rhetoric of war misleadingly suggests that cells or viruses have intentions, plans, strategies, or tactics, which are crucial to war. It disregards the fact that the biological process going on in our bodies lacks intentionality. Even Darwin recognized that what he called natural selection is "blind." There is no mastermind behind the biological process, and chance plays a crucial role in it. It is hence problematic to say that war metaphors are biologically grounded. It is much more the other way round: we project war metaphors to the realm of biology to make sense of biological processes by anthropomorphizing them.

Healthcare Professionals as Heroes on the Frontlines

Second, healthcare professionals are not soldiers any more than patients are, even though they are of course important agents in responding to the pandemic. Doctors practice agency in making vital decisions about treatment and care, and researchers around the world are key agents in the joint endeavor to develop tests, drugs, and vaccines. But what healthcare professionals practice is care, not war. Tuomas Forsberg (2020) asserts that in the pandemic "the task is to save lives which is one crucial dimension in warfare, too." There is a decisive difference, however: while doctors are committed to the universal right to care, in war only some lives are considered worth saving. As Elena Couceiro and María del Vigo (2020) have pointed out, universal access to healthcare is essential to what *peace* is about.

Applied to healthcare professionals, the narrative of war becomes a narrative of *heroism*. It casts doctors and nurses in the role of heroes who risk their lives to save lives. Even though this narrative is often intended to express gratitude, it imposes unreasonable expectations on healthcare professionals. As Jonathan Marron et al. (2020) argue, the heroization of health workers is problematic because few of them "entered their field anticipating risking their lives" as do soldiers who enlist voluntarily to war, and it is unfair to expect them to be war heroes no matter what their level of vulnerability and family situation. Similarly, Rachel Clarke (2020) writes that "classical heroes choose to put themselves in danger," they "aren't scared," "don't cry," are "immune to PTSD," "don't need work-life balance and lunch breaks," and "don't lie awake at night worrying about infecting their partners and children," whereas health workers "are highly skilled professionals who never volunteered to die for our country and should be as appropriately paid, trained and protected from industrial injury as anyone else."

The narrative of war is used as a *legitimizing discourse*. Wars inevitably have casualties; wars require sacrifices. The narrative of war heroism justifies putting health workers at risk and often at minimum wage. They are expected to sacrifice their lives in a war that the *nation* is waging against the common enemy. This nationalist discourse of war distracts us from structural inequalities, including the high exposure of low-paid women to the virus (Bateman & Ross, 2020; Booth, 2020). As Clarke (2020) says, the way health workers are offered "medals, memorials and flypasts increasingly feels like a clever and calculated distraction" from the fact that, in the United Kingdom, two-thirds of nurses are on minimum wage and the government initially failed to provide them with appropriate protective equipment: "The dehumanising narrative of healthcare as heroism benefits political leaders by deflecting attention from their dismal failure to keep staff from avoidable harm." It is disrespectful to treat healthcare professionals as soldiers because, throughout history, soldiers have been seen as expendable instruments that can be sacrificed for a greater cause.

Patients, Not Soldiers

Third, the narrative of war has been widely used in the media to cast patients in the role of soldiers battling COVID-19. This is problematic because it implies that those who survive fought so hard that they made it, and those who failed to survive are losers whose fighting spirit was not strong enough. Even when we do not explicitly think that psychological traits determine who survives, the language of battle easily leads us to such assumptions. When Johnson was treated for COVID-19 in intensive care, Trump (2020c) declared that Johnson will be fine because he is such a "strong person": "Strong. Resolute. Doesn't quit. Doesn't give up." The implication is clear: those who "lose the battle" are quitters, weak persons who simply give up.

The same problem pertains to using the language of war in depicting cancer patients as warriors or fighters. This has been criticized since Susan Sontag's (1978) influential *Illness as Metaphor*, but the narrative of battle still remains the dominant way of talking about cancer. I knew this is problematic, but I realized it in a concrete, embodied way only after I was diagnosed with breast cancer in May 2019 and immediately faced the narrative of battle.

"Now you just have to fight hard," I was told, time and again, and praised for how hard I was fighting.

The cancer itself did not feel like anything, which is typical in the early stages of cancer. It is the grueling treatments that make you feel ill, so it was difficult to understand what exactly I was supposed to battle against. For me, the main issue was anxiety about a possible lost future—fear of not seeing my children grow up. It was also difficult to deal with the *normative optimism* that was so prevalent in my surroundings, in the pink breast cancer culture— the overwhelming pressure to be positive (Meretoja, 2023b). It became very clear to me that the preferred cultural narrative is the one of waging a war on cancer with courage and optimism as if one could be healed by just having the right attitude and enough willpower.

And yet there is no research to suggest that a strong fighting spirit would help to defeat either coronavirus or cancer. In fact, research indicates the opposite: military metaphors harm cancer patients (Hauser & Schwarz, 2020). Those who recover from cancer or COVID-19 are fortunate but should not be praised for a successful battle anymore than those who die should be blamed for not fighting hard enough. Survival depends on access to treatment and on biological mechanisms, such as the immune system, not on psychological traits, such as courage, optimism, or fighting spirit.

But this is not the story people want to hear. In her analysis of what she calls disruptive breast cancer stories, Emilia Nielsen (2019) concludes that people generally do not want to hear stories of anger or grief although they are valuable in making room for a wider range of emotions linked to the experience of cancer. I would add that people generally do not want to hear stories of illness that end in death or stories in which it is not up to us whether we survive or not. We are used to the idea that good stories have heroes, and stories of blind biological mechanisms have no proper heroes. In fact, death or survival in war, too, is, at least for common soldiers at the frontline, more or less up to random chance. In popular war stories, however, heroism plays a crucial role—in them, soldiers are agents whose courage and cleverness make all the difference. When patients are compared to soldiers in battle, it is precisely to emphasize the significance of courage and toughness as factors crucial for survival.

In pandemic times, we are all potential patients and are urged to prepare for the fight by keeping ourselves fit and healthy. This is another way of overplaying the power of individual agency and distracting us from structural inequalities such as the exposure of lowest-income workers to the virus.

Narratives are a way of ascribing agency to patients by suggesting not only that they can affect the course of their illness but also that they have a causative role in bringing about their own illness.

Humans have a strong need to ascribe agency when things go wrong. It creates an illusion of control by suggesting that the catastrophe only affects people who have not taken the appropriate steps to stay safe—people who failed to be strong and alert soldiers in the war against the invisible enemy. This applies again to both cancer and COVID-19: a healthy lifestyle and alertness are supposed to make us invulnerable. It can feel reassuring to think that most COVID patients have "underlying health conditions" and many of them less than optimal lifestyles, such as smoking or obesity. After his own experience of falling ill with COVID-19, Johnson (2020b) attributed his illness to "a very common underlying condition. My friends, I was too fat," and he urged the British people to lose weight in the fight against the pandemic.

Nevertheless, the truth is that life is fragile, and we are all vulnerable: both cancer and COVID-19 can hit anyone. I had no known risk factors and yet got a cancer diagnosis at a young age, completely out of the blue. It made me realize how much my life was governed by an illusion of control. I had thought that if I keep myself superfit, eat a healthy diet, have children young, breastfeed them for over a year each, and so on, nothing could go this wrong. And yet the cells started to divide in my breast uncontrollably. When I got the cancer diagnosis, I could not help wondering what caused the cancer: Was there something I could have done differently, and was there some link to environmental issues—had I been exposed to some toxic chemicals? It is impossible to know. Oncologists told me that most cancers happen due to random cell mutation, independent of any lifestyle factors. It is simply bad luck. With COVID-19, too, some previously healthy people get seriously ill and die, and it has been hard to learn to live with this fundamental uncertainty. The narrative of war obscures this uncertainty and suggests that it is up to us whether we will stay safe or fall ill and die.

Joseph Grady (1997) has analyzed how the metaphor of fighting illness is based on the "primary metaphor" of "difficulties are opponents" which indicates "that not only verbal disagreements and arguments but any kind of action or process where we have trouble achieving our goals can be conceptualized as a fight": "Such a mapping might be directly motivated by the experience of frustration and exertion when we physically struggle with another person, a primary scene all of us have experienced as babies, if not more recently" (p. 167). As Elena Semino (2021) puts it, "Aggressive military powers and invaders are the most extreme examples of opponents, and wars are the most extreme examples of dealing with them." I would say that this is precisely the problem—there may be aspects of a struggle in dealing with illness and many other life challenges, but it is one step further to frame the struggle as *war*. Not all struggle is violent—there are also nonviolent struggles, although they tend to be downplayed even in cultural memory studies, as if violence were worth remembering at the cost of non-violence (see, e.g., Reading & Katriel, 2015). Struggling can be a complex process that is not necessarily a fight with an external enemy: it can be an internal struggle or a struggle with the challenges inherent in a certain life situation. A war has a clear beginning and end, and the metaphor suggests that illness can be vanquished by the right combat strategy, so it is particularly ill-equipped for thinking about long-term illnesses that do not involve a swift recovery and about their complex social aspects.

It is a broader problem with the vocabulary and narrative imagination around illness and health that we tend to think of them in dichotomous terms. There is insufficient awareness of how illness and health permeate each other: no one is always healthy, and ill people can also have much health in them.[7] With COVID-19, the symptoms caused by the infection are mild for most patients, but they are often accompanied by fear and anxiety (e.g., about infecting others unknowingly) and many suffer from long-term health complications. For many, social isolation and ongoing uncertainty are also major challenges. Overall, the narrative of war does not allow us to make sense of the complex social and psychological issues linked to the experience of going through COVID-19.

Not a Collective War Effort

Fourth, we are collectively crucial agents in the effort to curb the pandemic and deal with its aftermath, but just because this is a joint effort does not make it a war effort, and the agency it involves can be narrated in many different ways. The analogy of war is misplaced for numerous factual reasons, ranging from the impact of war and pestilence on the economy and the movement of goods and people (Edgerton, 2020) to crucial differences between the sensory experience of an armed conflict and the pandemic

---

[7] On health-within-illness, see Carel, 2008.

(Fairbanks, 2020). Resorting to the narrative of war means missing the opportunity to confront the complexity and specificity of the pandemic as a global crisis. It blinds us to the uniqueness of the social, psychological, and economic challenges it engenders. But even more serious than factual differences is that the narrative of war misses the opportunity to cultivate an alternative pandemic imagination imbued with a different kind of sense of agency and its limits—one that is critical of narrative mastery and an illusion of control. Some of the key problems in ascribing us the agency of soldiers include the following. First, it is an undemocratic type of agency; second, it is divisive and nationalist; third, it does not encourage us to take collective responsibility for the future; and fourth, it does not expand but rather diminishes our sense of the possible.

First, the language of war presents citizens as soldiers who follow orders from military leaders. This is a profoundly undemocratic way of framing the situation. Unsurprisingly, populist and authoritarian leaders have been particularly eager to use the rhetoric of war. For example, Ugandan President Yoweri Kaguta Museveni asserted: "During a war, you don't insist on your freedom. You willingly give it up in exchange for survival. During a war, you don't complain of hunger. . . . Let's obey and follow the instructions of the authorities" (Chenoy, 2020). It is interesting that particularly macho-style male leaders (such as Trump and Johnson) have resorted to the narrative of war, while female leaders have generally avoided it.[8] One reason may be the lack of a tradition—and concomitant narrative imagination—of female war heroes in which women political leaders might be tempted to place themselves and which would set narrative models for them, but other notable reasons include a commitment to the core values of democratic citizenship and international collaboration. Cultural differences are important, too (see Meretoja, 2023a). The narrative of war has been particularly popular in countries (such as the United States and the United Kingdom) in which the cultural memory of World War II has the positive connotation of a collective effort that led to victory. Due to their Nazi past, Germans, in contrast, are more aware than most countries of the dangers in military metaphors, and they harbor less romantic views of war as a collective effort that leads to a positive outcome. The German President Frank-Walter Steinmeier said early on that the pandemic is not a war but a "test of our humanity" (Carter, 2019).

---

[8] The study by Dada et al. (2021) shows that male political leaders "largely used [war metaphors] with greater volume and frequency."

In contrast to most world leaders, Chancellor Angela Merkel consistently addressed the pandemic with an explicit emphasis on the key values of democratic citizenship, starting from the choice of address in her televised speech (March 18, 2020), "Fellow citizens," and articulating how the pandemic has made clear a shared vulnerability which requires joint, democratic action based on shared knowledge:

> That is the message an epidemic brings home—how vulnerable we all are, how much we depend on the considerate behaviour of others and, ultimately, how, through joint action, we can protect ourselves and offer one another encouragement and support. . . . We are a democracy. We thrive not because we are forced to do something, but because we share knowledge and encourage active participation. This is a historic task, and it can only be mastered if we face it together. (Merkel, 2020)

As Ian Beacock (2020) puts it, Merkel "shrewdly sensed that the outbreak presents an opportunity for democratic strengthening" and provided a model for how to respond to "an era of interlinked and irresolvable global crises," such as those revolving around climate and unchecked capitalism.

Second, the narrative of war is a divisive, violent, and nationalist narrative that turns people and nations against each other. It involves comparisons of how well different nations have done in the war against the virus. Countries have been grouped into winners and losers, with charts of the vaccine race showing which countries have succeeded in vaccinating their population most rapidly. The narrative of war is typically used in a nationalist context, as a call to arms. It calls for sacrifices that are "not for each other, as fellow citizens and subjects of care, but for the nation" (Beacock, 2020). It is addressed to a nation, to a people, to build unity against a joint enemy. Queen Elizabeth asked the people "to take pride" in the British response to the crisis, even though humility would seem a more appropriate response. Such a nationalist narrative of pride is particularly dangerous given that the pandemic shows precisely that international collaboration is needed to curb the virus. It was never enough to vaccinate one country—a high enough percentage of the entire humankind needed to be vaccinated before an end was in sight for the global health emergency. Here, again, we should judge the situation from the perspective of future generations who will remember the decisions made and evaluate whether principles of justice and fairness were followed: "Let's not kid ourselves, the question of who gets which vaccine in the world will of course leave new wounds and new memories" because those who received help and those who were left behind will remember (Merkel, 2021).

Third, the pandemic is not just something that happens randomly—scientists generally agree that it is a result of human actions and political decisions in a way similar to global warming. The pandemic is not an inevitable natural disaster but is inextricably linked to how humans have systematically exploited animals and are exerting increasing pressure on the biosphere. Even if it is not absolutely certain whether the pandemic originated in wet markets where live animals are stacked one upon another, scientists know that these markets create ideal conditions for viruses to jump from one species to another. Scientists agree that global warming and deforestation have made conditions more favorable to pandemics as animals are forced to move to new habitats and come into contact with new species.[9] The pandemic shows that exploitation of the biosphere has consequences that we do not control as well as we think. We cannot change the past, but we can affect the future, and we should take collective responsibility by learning to respect non-human nature and our fundamental dependency on it. Dominant narratives of the pandemic have not focused enough on the lessons we should learn from it for the future—for example, we could learn about the limits of our agency and about our fundamental connectedness. Some consider the narrative of war empowering, but I would say that it gives a false sense of power. To take responsibility for the pandemic, from the perspective of future generations, it would be much more important to learn humility and learn about the limits of our agency.

Fourth, narratives are not only accounts of what has happened; they also open up possibilities. How does the narrative of war affect our sense of the possible, that is, our ability to imagine different routes to different futures and our sense of how things could be otherwise? If we fixate ourselves on the war narrative, we miss crucial possibilities precisely concerning the future—opportunities of cultivating a new kind of narrative imagination. I will conclude with some thoughts on these possibilities.

---

[9] For a discussion of the environmental root causes of the pandemic, see, e.g., Bernstein, 2020; Calas et al., 2020.

An Alternative Narrative of a Historical Crossroads

Instead of narrating the pandemic as a story of war, we could narrate it as a narrative of historical crossroads. Originally, *crisis* meant, as a medical term, the crossroads in which a patient reaches a decisive point of taking the road toward either recovery or death. We could narrate the pandemic and its aftermath as a still open-ended story of a point in history in which humankind faces the opportunity to choose between routes to different futures. In a way, we are always at such a crossroads, but this time there is a real potential for change because we have seen that people can change their behaviors and habits if there is enough sense of urgency. As Rebecca Solnit (2020) puts it, "things that were supposed to be unstoppable stopped, and things that were supposed to be impossible—extending workers' rights and benefits, freeing prisoners, moving a few trillion dollars around in the US—have already happened." The experience of being cut off from the flow of one's usual routines can have existential significance. It is an opportunity to reflect on one's priorities and values. Like a cancer diagnosis, the pandemic could be seen as a wake-up call for humanity—a moment of standing at a crossroads where we need to wake up and reflect on what really matters and decide which path to choose now. A narrative of a historical crossroads could make salient the possibility we now face, in the aftermath of the pandemic, to develop new forms of solidarity based on a more acute understanding of how we are fundamentally dependent on one another as inhabitants of a shared planet.

It is too simple to reduce a complex phenomenon, such as the pandemic, to any simple, concrete thing, as metaphors typically do by drawing an analogy between an abstract "target domain" and a concrete "source domain." Semino (2021) suggests that fire is an apt metaphor for the pandemic, but to my mind it is too simple and misleading in many ways. For example, it portrays the pandemic as a natural phenomenon, as one of the four basic elements, although in reality the pandemic is linked, in complex ways, to human action and policies of exploiting and destroying (non-human) nature. Narratives have more space for complexity than single metaphors. A narrative of being at a historical crossroads, for example, understood as a moment that calls for an existential awakening, could address the complexity of the fundamental questions concerning the direction in which humankind is heading. These are questions that have no simple answers. It is often a mark of productive narratives that they enrich our sense of the complexity of our most fundamental questions rather than provide answers to them. They open a space for ethical inquiry rather than preach a given doctrine.[10]

I am thinking of narratives that cultivate a sense of the pandemic as a lesson on the limits of our agency: on how we are not only agents but also sufferers; we not only affect but are also being affected, and often by forces that are beyond our control. We are at a crossroads that calls us to reflect on how our shared interdependency and destructibility are fundamental to the human condition—and something worth embracing. Agency is not only about autonomy and control but also about the ability to respond to others, to care about them, and to receive care and affection (Meretoja, 2023a, 2023b). We could move from an illusion of control to embracing our ability to connect, to depend on and draw strength from one another, which is a crucial ability, especially at times of global crises.

Cultivating a narrative imagination that holds open this possibility could help us imagine a society that acknowledges our interdependency as its central premise. Such imagination problematizes the neoliberal idea of self-sufficient, invulnerable individuals who are in full control of their lives. In the aftermath of the pandemic, we could seize the opportunity to build a new "narrative in-between," an intersubjective space in which a new global awareness of our mutual dependency gives rise to a new sense of solidarity across differences—solidarity between people, nations, different groups, communities, and species—which could help us build a more socially and environmentally just world for future generations.[11] When Merkel (2020) talks about the pandemic teaching us "how vulnerable we all are," she contributes to such narrative of learning together from this global crisis in order to take collective action to build a better future. Similarly, Arundhati Roy (2020) contributes to such narrative imaginary by describing the pandemic as a "portal" to a new world, and Solnit (2020) by delineating how a "new awareness of how each of us belongs to the whole and depends on it may strengthen the case for meaningful climate action, as we learn that sudden and profound change is possible after all."

The analysis in this chapter has drawn attention to a particular danger of narratives that we use to make sense of the world. Narratives tend to simplify reality by positioning humans or human-like agents as the ones who are in control of the world by acting upon it. Thereby narratives risk blinding us to

---

[10] On narratives that function as a form of ethical inquiry, see Meretoja, 2018, pp. 133–142.
[11] On the notion of the narrative in-between, see Meretoja, 2018, pp. 117–125.

the way in which reality consists in complex processes that evade the control of individual agents and that involve entangled networks of human and non-human agents. It is usually assumed that a sense of control is unequivocally a good thing. However, waking up to a realization that we have lived in an illusion of control can also be a highly valuable experience that can teach humility and cultivate a sense of connectedness.

So far there is little evidence of humankind learning anything much from the pandemic or taking a different course—and it now looks quite unlikely that anything like that will happen. But narratives are not only about what has happened or will in all likelihood happen. They also *hold open possibilities*. In the current moment of interconnected global crises, there is an urgent need for narratives that hold open the possibility we still have to leave behind an unsustainable way of life and imagine a world based on solidarity, care, and a sense of connection. The narrative of the crossroads is not a grand narrative that provides some kind of narrative mastery or false hope. It does not suggest that things will turn out fine. It merely makes visible the possibility that has opened for humankind. Narratives are not only retrospective accounts of what has happened, nor is their prospective dimension merely about narrating what is likely to happen. Narratives also open a space for imagining what is not yet but could be one day.[12] A narrative of a historical crossroads invites us precisely to such imagining of alternative futures and could make us more keenly aware of the stakes of our narrative imaginaries. It may be that some are already turning to retrospective narratives of lost possibilities, but the aftermath of the crisis, as a time of reflection, should involve looking both backward and forward: learning from what we have been through and imagining the post-pandemic world to come.

References

Andrews, M. (2014). *Narrative imagination and everyday life*. Oxford University Press.

Bateman, N., & Ross, M. (2020). Why has COVID-19 been especially harmful for working women? Brookings. October 2020. https://www.brookings.edu/essay/why-has-covid-19-been-especially-harmful-for-working-women/

Banjeglav, T., & Moll, N. (2021). Outbreak of war memories? Historical analogies of the 1990s wars in discourses about the coronavirus pandemic in Bosnia and Herzegovina and Croatia. *Southeast European and Black Sea Studies 21*(3), 353–372.

---

[12] On the not-yet aspect of narrative, see Andrews's (2014) discussion of narrative imagination.

Beacock, I. (2020). Germany gets it. *The New Republic*, April 1, 2020. https://newrepublic. com/article/157112/germany-gets-coronavirus

Bernstein, A. (2020). Coronavirus, climate change, and the environment. https://www. hsph.harvard.edu/c-change/subtopics/coronavirus-and-climate-change/

Biden, J. (2021). Biden signs executive orders for covid response. *New York Times*. January 22, 2021. https://www.nytimes.com/live/2021/01/21/us/joe-biden

Bleakley, A. (2017). *Thinking with metaphors in medicine: The state of the art*. Routledge.

Booth, R. (2020). Low-paid women in UK at "high risk of coronavirus exposure." *The Guardian*. March 29, 2020. https://www.theguardian.com/world/2020/mar/29/low-paid-women-in-uk-at-high-risk-of-coronavirus-exposure

Brockmeier, J. (2015). *Beyond the archive: memory, narrative, and the autobiographical process*. Oxford University Press.

Brockmeier, J., & Meretoja, H. (2014). Understanding narrative hermeneutics. *Storyworlds*, 6(2), 1–27.

Calas, J., Legassy, L., & Espagne, E. (2020). Pandemics: the environmental origins of COVID-19. Ideas for Development (iD4D) blog coordinated by Agence Française de Développement. https://ideas4development.org/en/pandemics-environmental-orig ins-covid-19/

Carel, H. (2008). *Illness*. Routledge.

Carter, L. (2019). Germany's president calls for patience, solidarity in face of pandemic. *Deutsche Welle*. April 11, 2019. https://www.dw.com/en/germanys-president-calls-for-patience-solidarity-in-face-of-pandemic/a-53095804

Chenoy, A. (2020). Why populist leaders use war rhetoric for all things related to the COVID-19 Pandemic. *The Wire*. August 19, 2020. https://thewire.in/politics/covid-19-war-militarism-public-health-populist-leaders

Clarke, R. (2020). Forget medals and flypasts—what we want is proper pay and PPE. *The Guardian*. May 2, 2020. https://www.theguardian.com/society/2020/may/02/nhs-doc tor-forget-medals-and-flypasts-what-we-want-is-proper-pay-and-ppe

Couceiro, E., & Vigo, del M. (2020). Covid-19: we are not soldiers. *Women's International League for Peace and Freedom*. March 25, 2020. https://www.wilpf.org/covid-19-we-are-not-soldiers/

Dada, S. Ashworth, H., Bewa M. J., & Dhatt, R. (2021 Jan). Words matter: Political and gender analysis of speeches made by heads of government during the COVID-19 pandemic. *BMJ Global Health* 6:e003910.

Edgerton, D. (2020). Why the coronavirus crisis should not be compared to the Second World War. *The New Statesman* April 3, 2020. https://www.newstatesman.com/science-tech/2020/04/why-coronavirus-crisis-should-not-be-compared-second-world-war

Fairbanks, E. (2020). The pandemic is not a war. *Huffington Post*. April 13, 2020. https:// www.huffpost.com/entry/war-pandemic-coronavirus-covid-19_n_5e90d449c5b67 2672149e1fa

Fernandes, S. (2017). *Curated stories: The uses and misuses of storytelling*. Oxford University Press.

Forsberg, T. (2020). Waging war against coronavirus: COVID-19 and the pandemic of metaphors. In *Multidisciplinary perspectives on the COVID-19 pandemic* (pp. 24–27). Helsinki Collegium for Advanced Studies.

Freeman, M. (2015). Narrative hermeneutics. In J. Martin, J. Sugarman, & K. L. Slaney (Eds.), *The Wiley handbook of theoretical and philosophical psychology* (pp. 234–247). Wiley Blackwell.

Gadamer, H.-G. (1984). The hermeneutics of suspicion. In G. Shapiro & A. Sica (Eds.), *Hermeneutics: Questions and prospects* (pp. 54–65). University of Massachusetts Press.

Grady, J. (1997). *Foundations of meaning: Primary metaphors and primary scenes* [Unpublished doctoral dissertation]. University of California at Berkeley.

Hauser, D. J., & Schwarz, N. (2020 Nov). The war on prevention II: Battle metaphors undermine cancer treatment and prevention and do not increase vigilance. *Health Commun, 35*(13), 1698–1704.

Husserl, E. (2006). *Späte Texte über Zeitkonstitution (1929– 1934). Die C-Manuskripte.* Springer.

Johnson, B. (2020a). Coronavirus: "We must act like any wartime government." BBC News. March 17, 2020. https://www.bbc.com/news/av/uk-51936760

Johnson, B. (2020b). Boris Johnson: Read the prime minister's keynote speech in full. October 6, 2020. https://www.conservatives.com/news/2020/boris-johnson--read-the-prime-minister-s-keynote-speech-in-full

Macron, E. (2020). "We are at war": France imposes lockdown to combat virus. *Reuters.* March 17, 2020. https://www.reuters.com/video/watch/idOVC5B4U2P

Mäkelä, M., & Meretoja, H. (2022), Critical approaches to the storytelling boom. *Poetics Today, 43*(2), 191–218.

Marron, J., Dizon, D., Symington, B., Thompson, M., and Rosenberg, A. (2020). Waging war on war metaphors in cancer and COVID-19. *JCO Oncology Practice* 16(10), 624–627. Martínez García, A. (2021). Memories of war and the COVID-19 crisis in Spain. *Hu Arenas 4,* 366–378.

Meretoja, H. (2014). *The narrative turn in fiction and theory: The crisis and return of storytelling from Robbe-Grillet to Tournier.* Palgrave Macmillan.

Meretoja, H. (2018). *The ethics of storytelling: Narrative hermeneutics, history, and the possible.* Oxford University Press.

Meretoja, H. (2020). Stop narrating the pandemic as a story of war. *Open Democracy.* May 19, 2020. https://www.opendemocracy.net/en/transformation/stop-narrating-pandemic-story-war/

Meretoja, H. (2021). A dialogic of counter-narratives. In K. Lueg & M. Wolff Lundholt (Eds.), *Routledge handbook of counter-narratives* (pp. 30–42). Routledge.

Meretoja, H. (2023a). Implicit narratives and narrative agency: Evaluating pandemic storytelling. *Narrative Inquiry 33*(2), 288–316.

Meretoja, H. (2023b). Hermeneutic awareness in uncertain times: Post-truth, narrative agency, and existential diminishment. In H. Meretoja & M. Freeman (Eds.), *The use and abuse of stories: New directions in narrative hermeneutics* (pp. 55–85). Oxford University Press.

Merkel, A. (2020). An address to the nation by Federal Chancellor Merkel. March 18, 2020. https://www.bundesregierung.de/breg-de/themen/coronavirus/statement-chancellor-1732296

Merkel, A. (2021). Coronavirus: Angela Merkel warns Davos against vaccine race. January 26, 2021. https://www.dw.com/en/coronavirus-angela-merkel-warns-davos-against-vaccine-race/a-56348151

NHS. (2020). NHS army of volunteers to start protecting vulnerable from coronavirus in England. 7 April 2020. https://www.england.nhs.uk/2020/04/nhs-volunteer-army-now-ready-to-support-even-more-people/

Nielsen, E. (2019). *Disrupting breast cancer narratives: Stories of rage and repair.* University of Toronto Press.

Reading, A., & Katriel, T. (2015). Introduction. In A. Reading & T. Katriel (Eds.), *Cultural memories of non-violent struggles* (pp. 1–35). Palgrave Macmillan.

Ricoeur, P. (1992). *Oneself as another.* Translated by K. Blamey. University of Chicago Press.

Roy, A. (2020). The pandemic is a portal. *Financial Times.* April 3, 2020.

Semino, E. (2021). "Not soldiers but fire-fighters"—Metaphors and Covid-19. *Health Commun, 36*:1,50–58.

Solnit, R. (2020). "The impossible has already happened": What coronavirus can teach us about hope. *The Guardian.* April 7, 2020. https://www.theguardian.com/world/2020/apr/07/what-coronavirus-can-teach-us-about-hope-rebecca-solnit

Sontag, S. (1978). *Illness as metaphor.* Farrar, Straus & Giroux.

Trump, D. (2020a). "Invisible enemy": Trump says he is "wartime president" in coronavirus battle – video. *The Guardian.* March 23, 2020. https://www.theguardian.com/world/video/2020/mar/23/invisible-enemy-trump-says-he-is-wartime-president-in-coronavirus-battle-video

Trump, D. (2020b). Trump says coronavirus worse "attack" than Pearl Harbor. *BBC.* May 7, 2020. https://www.bbc.com/news/world-us-canada-52568405

Trump, D. (2020c). Trump on Boris Johnson being taken into intensive care: "He's been really something very special; strong, resolute, doesn't quit, doesn't give up. *Twitter,* @ *washingtonpost* Apr 7, 2020.

Wilkinson, A. (2020). Pandemics are not wars. *Vox.* April 15, 2020. https://www.vox.com/culture/2020/4/15/21193679/coronavirus-pandemic-war-metaphor-ecology-microbiome

Wise, J. (2020). How the coronavirus could take over your body (before you ever feel it). *New York Magazine.* March 19, 2020. https://nymag.com/intelligencer/2020/03/the-story-of-a-coronavirus-infection.html

6

Beyond Trauma Narratives

How the Military Siege of Sarajevo (1992–1995) Shaped
Stories Told in the Aftermath

Luka Lucić and Guro Nore Fløgstad

Continuous sociocultural disruptions caused by the outbreak of the coronavirus pandemic are bewildering. Prolonged quarantines, social distancing,
sudden work and school interruptions all affect how we experience space
and time, two basic categories constitutive of human lived experience. Yet,
amid the increasing need to come to terms with novel spatial and temporal
boundaries shaped by the pandemic, perhaps the most difficult to conceptu-
alize and predict are the long-term effects of such spatio-temporal changes
on young people. How do widespread changes and transformations of activities affect the way young people make sense and make meaning of their
situated experience? And how will disruptions caused by the pandemic affect
how they think and feel in the aftermath of the acute crisis? To better understand these questions amid the global crisis caused by the coronavirus
outbreak, we analyze narratives from a more "minor" and regional crisis
that started three decades earlier. By examining narratives written by adults
who, as children, lived through the four-year-long military siege of Sarajevo
(1992–1995)—a period during which the categories of space and time were
also radically redefined—we seek to offer a lens that can help us make sense
of the effects that current conditions of radical change have on the psychological development of young people. In this work, we define *conditions of
radical change* as prolonged sociocultural circumstances in which space and
time abruptly and suddenly compress, expand, or otherwise meaningfully
change, thereby perforce transforming human activities.

When examining the effects of crises, psychology tends to emphasize
terminal conditions. An overwhelming majority of contemporary psychological research into conditions of radical change—such as war, urban destruction, pandemic, and environmental disasters—actively looks for the

Luka Lucić and Guro Nore Fløgstad, *Beyond Trauma Narratives* In: *Narrative in Crisis*. Edited by: Martin Dege and Irene
Strasser, Oxford University Press. © Oxford University Press 2024. DOI: 10.1093/oso/9780197751756.003.0006

effects of trauma, emotional damage, and delays across normative developmental processes experienced in the aftermath. Recently—almost as quickly
as the virus itself—the narrative that the coronavirus pandemic has triggered,
a worldwide mental-health crisis took hold (Ornstein et al., 2020; Solomon,
2020). Yet, when it comes to the psychological effects of crisis conditions,
data emerging from long-term epidemiological studies and meta-analyses of
clinical and psychological research point in a different direction. Specifically,
they show that depending on the specific context and exact nature of their
experience—between 10% and 45% of young people growing up amid the
conditions of war experience long-term anxiety, depression, or otherwise
show symptoms associated with posttraumatic stress disorder (PTSD) in the
aftermath (Attanayake et al., 2009; Fazel et al., 2005; Laor et al., 1997; Thabet
et al., 2002; for a review, see Peltonen & Punamäki, 2010). When examining
these data systematically, we face several glaring questions. The primary
one is: What happens to those 55–90% affected by war who do not develop
symptoms associated with trauma or PTSD in the aftermath? How do they
cope? Responding to such questions from the resilience perspective, study
after study demonstrates that most survivors either recover quickly or never
show a substantial decline in mental health (Bonanno, 2004). Similarly, recent data examining the effects of the coronavirus pandemic across 65
worldwide studies show that, by mid-2020, for most people, psychological
symptoms they may have developed at the onset of the pandemic decreased
and were comparable to pre-pandemic levels (Robinson et al., 2022).

   In response to the question, "How is life shaped beyond crisis experiences?,"
we offer a narrative analysis that attempts to complicate these frozen notions.
Maintaining that exposure to conditions of radical change leads to long-term
trauma or, alternatively, that resilience represents a distinct trajectory from
the process of recovery characterized by a positive emotional experience,
both homogenize a complex set of human reactions by reducing them to still
and embalmed categories. In contrast, we engage in the narrative analysis as
we try to understand the dynamic, malleable, culturally situated, and heterogeneous nature of human psychological processes that develop during—and
in response to—the conditions of radical change. Taking the sociocultural
approach—which teaches us that higher psychological functions initially
develop their social form and only subsequently do they become individual
(Vygotsky, 1934/1962)—in this work, we specifically examine narratives
written by 10 participants about their unique activities during the siege of
Sarajevo, the longest military blockade of a city in modern history. As we

describe spaces within the besieged city shaped by military destruction, we consider the range of unique activities these spaces afforded to the young people. Rather than focusing solely on the positive or the negative valence of their experience, our analyses aim to understand how such unique activities available during the 1,335-day-long siege—this is a full year longer than the siege of Leningrad during World War II—shaped the way our participants make sense and make meaning of their experiences. The 10 participants who contributed to this work grew up in Sarajevo, lived there during the siege, and continue to reside in the city.

To situate our analysis in the appropriate sociocultural context, we first describe the conditions of four-year-long military siege that our participants lived with and grew up during. Following this overview, we explain how contexts shaped by the siege enabled unique activities to emerge, before moving to analyze the narratives written by our participants. In line with sociocultural theory and contemporary research in developmental psychology (Cole, 1996; Daiute, 2010; Daiute & Lucić, 2010; Lucić, 2016; Luria, 1976; Rogoff, 2003; Vygotsky, 1934/1962; Zittoun, 2006), this work employs narrative analysis as a method to explore how various unique contexts rendered by the military siege continue to mediate thought processes of our participants in the aftermath of the acute crisis period. Theoretically, our research views language—employed as narrative—as a tool for imposing on experience some organized differentiation between action, cognition, and feeling, thereby making sense of that experience. By explicitly focusing our analysis in this work on the enactment of adverbs in narrative, we seek to understand how the activities of our participants during the siege shaped their developing thought processes. In our analysis, adverbs act as a magnifying lens. Adverbs function in syntax to modify or qualify verbs (or adjectives) to express a relation of place, time, circumstance, or, alternatively, to express the manner of action. Hence, the syntactic relevance that adverbs bear specifically on verbs allows us to understand how our participants—in the aftermath of the crisis—reflect on their activities during the acute siege period. More specifically, by analyzing the use of adverbs, we build on Labov and Waletzsky's (1967) narrative analysis scheme, which distinguishes two narrative functions, *evaluative* and *referential*, to argue that wartime activities in dangerous physical contexts motivate narrative thought processes to become increasingly more evaluative even long after the siege has ended. Our findings suggest a complex sociocognitive response to the crisis beyond the singular focus on trauma narratives or a quick return to normalcy.

Looking Through a Lens of a Regional Crisis: The Siege of Sarajevo

Considered to be the longest blockade of a city in modern military history, the siege of Sarajevo started gradually during the spring of 1992. Fueled by the resurgence of ethnonationalism across former Yugoslavia amid a sharp economic downturn, armed conflict swept across Bosnia and Herzegovina (Clark, 2014; Woodward, 1995). When the war erupted, it caught many Sarajevans by surprise. Less than a decade prior, this city projected a successful model of ethnic and religious integration into the world by hosting the 1984 Winter Olympic Games. But in May 1992, the flames across the city were not Olympic. When the initial barricades went up across the city center—used to prevent free movement of citizens and section off various city neighborhoods along ethnic lines—most thought that this extraordinary situation would last only a few days (see Figure 6.1). However, conditions quickly deteriorated. During the initial months of the conflict, the supply of

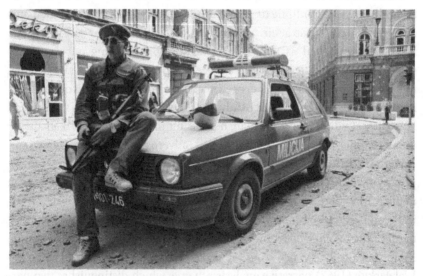

Figure 6.1 This photo taken during the spring of 1992 depicts one of Sarajevo's central areas, the square adjacent to Vječna Vatra during the early period of the siege. Central to the photo is a member of Territorial Defence under the command of General Jovan Divjak. During this time, the formal army was not yet present in the city, and local militias controlled the streets.
Source: Photo by Jordi Pujol Puente.

water, food, and electricity was strained and frequently interrupted. A curfew starting at 9 PM was imposed, and, with it, the city began to assume a gaunt, untidy look. Main roads and the majority of buildings were in poor repair, the streets at night were dimly lit for fear of military invasion, and the shops were mostly half-empty. Meat was scarce and milk practically unattainable; there was a shortage of coal, sugar, and petrol, and gradually a severe shortage of bread ensued. It would be months before the UN started delivering humanitarian assistance.

But it was in the fall of 1992, when the paramilitary units set up checkpoints on the barricades and the public transportation completely halted, that the situation inside of the besieged city became dire. During July and August, Serbian army troops, tanks, and cannons gradually replaced the militia on the barricades—occupying the suburbs—until every road leading in or out of the city was sealed. By September, approximately 300,000 citizens of Sarajevo were living under a full-blown military siege enforced by 13,000 occupying troops. Throughout the siege, the city experienced an average of 330 mortar shell impacts per day, resulting in immense destruction of the built environment. By the summer of 1993, virtually all of the buildings in Sarajevo were damaged, and more than 30,000 were destroyed (Figure 6.2) (Bassiouni, 1994).

Under the strain of new temporal and spatial conditions produced by the siege, prewar activities often changed or altered course to meet the new demands. Such changes were driven primarily by environmental destruction and the resulting transformation of everyday spaces such as family dwellings or public spaces (Maček, 2009; Pilav, 2020). As Pilav (2012) describes in her research, because of war, the overground city became an extremely dangerous, high-risk battlefield where the movement of civilians was reduced to a minimum. But the contraction of the space in the overground city resulted in its proportional expansion in the underground. Previously underutilized underground areas, such as basements and storage areas, became dynamic multirelational spaces where civilians spent a great deal of time. Sleeping, eating, playing, schooling, and socializing happened underground, where one was relatively safe from the artillery fire which was quickly reducing the overground city to rubble. But life under siege also brought with it entirely new and unexpected activities. Perhaps nothing symbolizes the harshness of this period more than the image of exhausted people with plastic jugs queuing for purified water in front of the Sarajevo Brewery. When the shortage of drinking water became acute, it forced Sarajevans to collect river

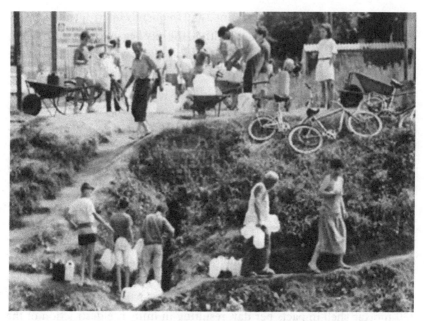

Figure 6.2 This photo taken at the height of the siege shows Sarajevans at the bank of the Miljacka River in the process of obtaining water. Bicycles and trolleys depticted in this photo became useful means of transporting water.

water from a shallow and quite polluted Miljacka River and then apply purification tablets to make it safe for drinking (see Figure 6.2). Long lines also formed to receive the food rationed from UN donations, and almost all of the trees in city parks were cut down to be used as heating sources.

Due to the widespread destruction of the urban environment as well as general shortages of food and water, the activities of 65,000 young people stranded in the besieged city oscillated between attempts to transform the war landscape into a context suitable for play (see Figure 6.3) and an intense struggle to acquire daily necessities (see Figure 6.4). A short narrative written by Edin—one of the 10 participants in this study—gives a glimpse into the daily activities of a 13-year-old boy during the early period of the siege. Referencing the Sarajevo War Tunnel—the only route in and out of the besieged city—in the first clause of his narrative and Sarajevo airport in the second clause, Edin writes,

Before the tunnel opened, you had to run across the runway. It was dangerous, but we had to cross in order to obtain food. As a boy, I was crossing

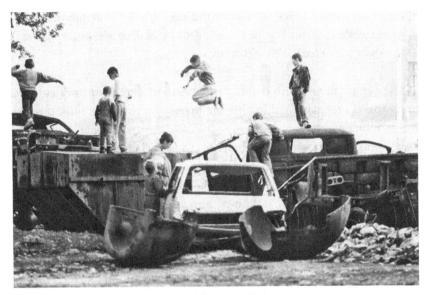

Figure 6.3 Jump! Destroyed automobiles were first piled on as a barricade, before becoming an active playground.
Source: Photo by Gervasio Sánchez.

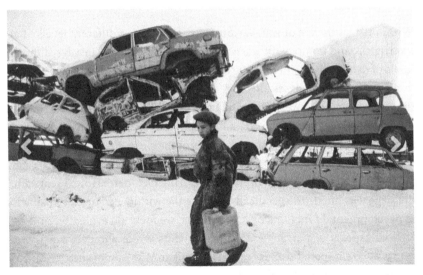

Figure 6.4 A young boy carries a canister of water over snow-covered streets during the winter of 1994.
Source: Photo by Enrico Dagnin.

the runway, and I risked my life for the soup powder, milk powder, etc. After a while, the tunnel opened, making life in Sarajevo a lot easier. I guess that's why it is called the Tunnel of Hope.

The danger involved in the described activity stands in stark contrast to its goals: a teenager risking his life to acquire soup and milk powder. But as Edin's narrative shows, this activity—like many others during the siege—was characterized by a heightened experience of space and time as he "had to" "run across the runway." Living amid a dangerous and fast-changing physical environment, he had to be attuned to space, understand how it changes, and know how to use it to merely get on with basic daily life. But Edin's narrative does not only focus on the referential aspects of his activity but also captures the more evaluative personal elements that become manifest during the times of heightened danger: the youth, danger, bewilderment, and the tumult one feels during the period of acute crisis, when "It was dangerous, but we had to . . . . As a boy, . . . I risked my life."

Analysis of Narratives: Adverbial and Attributive Adverbs

Within the landscape of war, various activities assume different levels of attentiveness and complexity, garner various interests, and involve different levels of danger. By distinguishing between adverbial and attributive adverbs in narratives, our analyses aim to reveal a within-person heterogeneity that the various spatial contexts that situate these activities produce. Seen from an individual vantage point, our data highlight that everyday activities, spread across multiple mutually exclusive spaces of the siege, structurally shape the stories participants tell in the aftermath. To illustrate this, we draw on narrative data collected with 10 individuals during October 2015, 20 years after the siege was lifted. To specifically explore the within-person heterogeneity of developmental functions beyond trauma, we focus on evaluative and referential aspects of narratives that participants wrote about two activities across different spatial contexts: (a) daily walk to War School and (b) journey through the Sarajevo War Tunnel.

The evaluative function in the narrative was first defined by Labov and Waletzsky (1967). According to their narrative analysis scheme, *evaluation* is generally juxtaposed with the referential function, which serves as a narrative core and is organized as canonical events that often involve scripted ways of accomplishing an activity. In contrast, the *evaluative function* serves to establish a point of personal interest for narrators in relation to their activities. As opposed to referential function, evaluation captures what those involved in the action—narrator as well as other characters in a narrative know—think, feel, believe, and desire. Evaluation offers the listener information about the narrator's point of view. In other words, it establishes the point of a narrative. Subsequent developmental research has strongly associated narrative evaluation with personal significance, interpretation, and signaling of the meaning-making and sense-making processes (Bruner & Haste, 1987; Daiute, 2010; Daiute & Nelson, 1997; Lucić, 2013; Nelson, 1985, 1996; Peterson & McCabe, 1983). In line with these studies our analyses will show that the more novel and precarious the space of the described activity is (such as a journey through the Sarajevo War Tunnel), the more evaluative the psychological processes between the self and the context of the activity are.

Our analyses of narratives are functional. While we consider *what* is told in the narrative, we primarily focus on *how* the narrative is told. Our work explores how various linguistic categories are used in their narratives to interweave and interlace the complex relationship of the developing persons' thought processes and their originating context. For example, by explicitly focusing on the linguistic category of prepositions, words that indicate the location (in, near, beside, on top of, etc.) or some other relationship between a noun or pronoun and other parts of the sentence, previous work by the first author shows that growing up amid war gives rise to referential thought processes that draw on spatial and temporal relations (see Lucić & Bridges, 2018). In the present work, we extend our analysis to include the category of adverbs. As a linguistic category, adverbs present a valuable unit of analysis because they can semantically serve as referential (e.g., to express temporal and spatial relations) and evaluative words (e.g., to express the manner of action).

Because adverbs function in syntax to modify or qualify an adjective or a verb to express a relation of place, time, circumstance (e.g., now, then, there, tomorrow, behind, down) or to express the manner of action (e.g., anxiously, boldly, fondly), the analysis of their use in narrative construction can yield information about participants' thought processes developmentally situated at the junction of their activities and their environmental contexts. In our analysis, we employ the language-specific distinction made in Bosnian grammar according to which adverbs are divided into two groups; *adverbial* and *attributive* (Jahić et al., 2000). Functionally similar to prepositions, *adverbial adverbs* are referential. They convey meanings such as tense or location and indicate place, time, or goal and typically take on a referential function more in line with prepositions. They modify the verb to indicate the place, time, cause, goal, or intent of the action. *Attributive adverbs*, on the other hand, include adverbs of manner and are evaluative. They indicate mode, characteristics, property, way of doing an action, or intensity and can often be classified as linguistic intensifiers. They rarely contribute to the referential meaning in a clause or a narrative but rather serve as evaluative devices. In our sample, attributive adverbs such as *dangerously, diligently, barely, somehow,* and *terribly* are employed by the narrators to qualify their actions in relation to the physical context and signal emotional undertone (such as confusion, bewilderment, surprise, awe, wonder) or express the personal significance of the actions that they modify and intensify.

The data employed in this study were thoroughly analyzed. First, the narratives were translated by two native speakers of both English and Bosnian. Second, to ensure analyzability and accountability of the data and make analysis possible for non-Bosnian speakers, the relevant data parts were glossed by a native speaker of Bosnian, according to the Leipzig Glossing Rules. Glossing involves using notational conventions (e.g., abbreviations) to provide information about the meanings and grammatical properties of words and word parts. Glossing can vary in detail depending on the audience and the methodological necessities. For this study, only words and constructions involving adverbs, both attributive and adverbial, were included in the glossing, as seen in examples (1) and (2) in Figure 6.5.

Seen through the prism of adverbs, narratives written 20 years following the conclusion of the hostilities show that when narrating about situations of heightened danger, individuals in the process of sense-making become attentive to the physical context within which their activities are situated and, at the same time, highly attuned to the relationship between the self and the spaces experienced. In the next section, we build on this methodology to show how a dynamic mind—a mind in the process of trying to understand—employs language to makes sense and makes meaning of the situated experience.

(1)
Subject 2: Adverbial uses, from War School day narrative

Iako	*mi*	*je*	*škola*	*bila*	*blizu,*	*tada*	*se*	*to*	*činilo*
even	me.OBJ	is	school	was	close.ADV	then.ADV	itself	it	seemed

'And even though the school was close by, it seemed'

kilometrima	*daleko.*
kilometers.ADV	away.ADV

'kilometers away.'

(2)
Subject 9: Attributive, from War Tunnel narrative

Tunel je bio	*dosta*	*nizak*	*i bilo je dosta*	*vlage*	*u njemu, ali je*
tunnel is was	a lot.ADV	low.ADJ	and was is a lot.ADV	moisture	in him but is

'The tunnel was quite low and there is a lot of moisture in it,'

meni	*kao*	*detetu*	*to*	*sve*	*bilo*	*interesantno.*
me	as	child	that	all	was	interesting.ADV

'but to me as a child it was all interesting.'

Figure 6.5 Analysis Example: Glossing using the Leipzig Rules, as shown in these examples, involves using notational conventions to provide information about the meanings and grammatical properties of words and word parts.

Activities in Space Are Enacted in Narrative

How do moments of crisis shape the stories we tell in the aftermath? As we analyze in more detail in this section, when young people tell stories about their activities reflecting on situations of heightened danger—such as a trip through the Sarajevo War Tunnel—their use of attributive adverbs increases compared to when the same participants narrate about more routine everyday activities, such as walking to school. On average, narratives written about the trip through the Sarajevo War Tunnel were 101.1 words long, while the narratives about the walk to school are shorter, running on average 68.1 words in length. Generally, narrative length is a good predictor of narrative complexity (Schwalm, 1985). When narrating about the Sarajevo War Tunnel, participants employ attributive adverbs on average every 18.42 words. Comparatively, in narratives about a walk to War School, they use attributive adverbs on average every 25.49 words. Closer inspection using a paired sample t-test shows that this difference is approaching significance $t(10) = -1.649$. $p = 0.066$, which we see as an important trend, especially considering that a very small sample was used for this analysis. In comparison, the difference in the use of adverbial adverbs across the two narrative contexts was not as pronounced, with participants employing adverbial adverbs on average every 53.86 words in the narratives about the Sarajevo War Tunnel and every 40.21 words on average in narratives about the daily walk to school.

In what follows, we delve deeper into our analysis by looking at the use of two types of adverbs across various contexts to illustrate their role as related to the narrator's thought processes. To do so, we use narrative responses written by one participant, Sena, who was 15 years old when the war broke out. At the time of the study, she was 38 years old and still living in Sarajevo. She narrates in response to a set of prompts that asked her to reflect on everyday activities across various spaces rendered by the siege. As the baseline assessment, we would like the readers to consider a narrative in which Sena describes a typical school day in Sarajevo before the war started. For the convenience of readers, we have bolded all **adverbs** but underlined only the <u>**attributive adverbs**</u> in the narrative. Moreover, to better contrast the referential and evaluative elements across the entire narrative, we have italicized all *prepositions and adverbs*. The reader can note all narrative aspects when they consider Sena's response to the narrative prompt "Write a letter to a person younger than yourself and in this letter to describe one day in Sarajevo before the war started."

> Days were all the same—carefree. Each day we would walk *back* home *from* school <u>*together*</u>. *Through* the main street, we went as a "pack." Smiling and discussing the school topics. We walked *next to* each shop *along* the way home. There we stopped. Everyone would *from* their <u>*neatly*</u> washed and ironed school uniforms (aprons) take *out* a coin, or two. We bought chocolates, sweets, and biscuits "Harmonija." We laughed and enjoyed the sweets. We were 8/2 class. Boys and girls, comrades.

Reading Sena's narrative, we get a sense that her childhood was characterized by carefree days that seemingly amalgamated into one. Running 83 words in length, her narrative consists mainly of nouns, verbs, and adjectives. Most verbs and adjectives employed by Sena have a positive valence (such as carefree, smiling, laughed, enjoyed), and a peaceful and pleasant attitude permeates the narratives. According to her account, prewar Sarajevo was a stimulating place for young people. Smiling as she visited the shops, Sena's walk home from school seems like a distant saunter through peaceful streets, an activity filled with joy, laughs, and sweets. Moreover, to contextualize the streets of prewar Sarajevo, she does not directly describe a specific situation. Instead, Sena portrays an expected state of the world and uses her narrative to create a bricolage that depicts a peaceful urban setting. Two adverbs that she employs in her narrative are attributive (*together*, *neatly*), and one is adverbial (*out*).

Like many Sarajevans, Sena could not anticipate that—only a few months following the events that she described above—the same streets would become a high-risk battlefield. Yet, even throughout such dangerous conditions, she and other young people continued engageing in activities that gave them some semblance of routine, such as attending school. However, the enormous shift in the context of such activities is reflected in Sena's narrative description of her journey to school during the war. Not only is the theme of her narrative different: as the city becomes more dangerous, the narrative structure begins to change, and adverbs start to appear more frequently across her response.

> Most school days passed as *through* the fog. And even though the school was *close* by, *then* it seemed kilometers *away*. Every time I went to school I feared that a shell would fall. *In* the center of town, *where* our apartment was located, there were no snipers but *instead* shells were falling around the clock. I went *on foot* and frequently it happened that we would be sent back *home* because the shelling started. The school was transferred *to* another building (**now** the building of BKC), and classes were held *in* the hallway. The classroom was improvised. We were *in* the hallway, sitting *in* chairs, and we kept books *on* our laps. The school was **then** held depending *on* whether or not there was electricity. I do not remember the feelings I had while we were sitting *there*, but the gap *in* knowledge remains *till* today. And four years of schooling (entire secondary school) no one can *ever* make up to me. There was no socializing, dates, cramming, school trips, skipping *from* classes. Nothing.

While situated and highly referential to her specific neighborhood, Sena's narrative helps to illustrate the realities of everyday life faced by the majority of young people living in Sarajevo during the siege. Comparing this narrative to the prior one, we notice several details directly relevant to our inquiry. First, this narrative response is 163 words long, almost twice as long as Sena's earlier narrative. Even though she starts her narrative by saying that *most school days passed as through the fog*, she goes to great lengths to describe—in detail—the changes that ensued in the context of her activities. In the second sentence, Sena employs three adverbs in succession *close, then, away* to alert the reader to a subjective/objective distinction in her experience of space and distance. Sena mentions that her school was *close by* because the location of her classroom changed: the school got closer. Throughout the besieged city— instead of the prewar school buildings—educational activities took place in informal, safe spaces. This is also why, later in her narrative, Sena mentions that: "the school was transferred *to* another building (**now** the building of BKC), and classes were held *in* the hallway." Multiple schooling locations were established within improvised locations across each neighborhood to minimize the risk students encountered in the dangerous overground city (for a detailed discussion on the reorganization of schooling during the siege, see Lucić, 2021). But even though the schooling location was objectively closer to her residence, subjectively, because of the danger from shelling and snipers, it seemed "kilometers *away*" to Sena.

Additionally, by examining how this narrative is told, we notice a prevalent emphasis on the space of her wartime activities. In addition to being infused with elements of a personal nature, such as the location of her apartment to the school, the feeling of the book on her lap while she sat in an improvised hallway classroom, many aspects of the narrative, such as the prepositions she frequently employs, are referential. Moreover, out of 11 adverbs that she employs, 8 are adverbial adverbs (such as *close, then, away*) used to modify the verb to indicate place, time, cause, goal, or intent of the action. Taken to- gether, prepositions and adverbial adverbs account for 19 out of 163 words or 12% of the entire response. Such a large percent of words used to directly introduce key spatial-relational and temporal information—information that situates the narrative and orients the reader through the narrated space and time—is one of the characteristics of narratives that directly address the satiations of radical change (Lucić, 2016; Lucić & Bridges, 2018).

From the literature on the relation between spatial language and thought, we know that conceptualizations are affected by cognition and experience. Moving in space—or even *thinking about* moving in space—are actions that affect our symbolic structures and conceptualization and, subsequently, linguistic expressions (Ramscar et al., 2010, for an overview). Experience affects language, simply put. When we engage in spatial thinking, we also affect our conceptual representations of space and, subsequently, the way we talk about them. While there is undoubtedly a lot more than spatial terms to analyze in this narrative, both from the perspective of the content and the form, examining the use of prepositions and adverbial adverbs leads us to characterize this narrative as highly referential. Comparing it to the prewar narrative, Sena shows an acute understanding of space and spatial changes that ensued with (or because) the onset of the siege. She describes how these changes impacted her activities. But perhaps because walking to a War School was a frequent activity, one that happened regularly during the siege, Sena does not appear bewildered or confused by spatial changes. She simply describes them, as a matter of fact.

Other activities upon which young people of Sarajevo embarked were often far more dangerous. Perhaps the most dangerous, anticipation-filled activity involved passing through the Sarajevo War Tunnel. Officially named Objekat Dobrinja–Butmir, this muddy and narrow underground passage functioned as a de facto lifeline, the only connection of a besieged city with the external world. Over the two and a half years of its existence, thousands of people passed through the tunnel. Sena was one of them. Asked to describe her trip through the tunnel, 20 years following the events of the siege, she writes,

> The tunnel, for me _**always**_ represented a mythical place _about_ which we talked in a low voice. Just getting _to_ the tunnel was a big deal. One summer _in_ the middle of the war I _**totally**_ "snapped" and said that I must go _to_ the seaside. I was _**maybe**_ 16–17 years old. _With_ my then-boyfriend, I made a plan to go to the island of Krk and stay _at_ his cousin's. And to this day I am _**not clear**_ how our parents allowed us to go. Parents _during_ the war, stop being parents. The family of my boyfriend organized the whole trip for us, a tarpaulin covered truck that transported us _to_ the tunnel and _from_ the tunnel. I was dying of fear _in_ that truck thinking that they will shoot at us. The tunnel itself was a little, common, dark and stuffy place. The _**hardest**_ thing was that the whole time I had to walk _**stooped**_ as low as I walked. My back was aching and I remember that I _**barely**_ weathered the effort. It was _**terribly**_ stuffy. It was _**hard**_ and the only thing I was thinking is that I could _**barely**_ wait for _when_ it would finish. _**Luckily**_ I didn't have a backpack _on_ my back because my boyfriend took it. I watched people in _front_ of me _**how**_ they themselves struggle _with_ things they are carrying.

When compared to the last two narratives also written by Sena, this description of the dangerous trip through the tunnel is both qualitatively and quantitatively different. First, it is 40% longer than the War School trip narrative and almost three times as long as the narrative about the prewar time. Here Sena uses 230 words to describe her journey. Similar to the description of the school trip, Sena uses 11 prepositions in her narrative, but this time only two adverbial adverbs. Together, these referential words account for 6% of her entire narrative as Sena orients the reader through the narrated space. However—when examining the tunnel narrative—we also notice the presence of narrative evaluation, a function that did not feature prominently in the two earlier narratives. The evaluative function is specifically evoked in this narrative by the high use of attributive adverbs.

While in the prior narrative Sena used only two, this time she employs 12 attributive adverbs, words such as *always, totally, not clear, barely,* and *terribly.* She does this to illustrate her feelings and impressions of the actions undertaken and explain the emotional significance of her actions. We recognize heightened evaluation in this narrative through such frequent use of attributive adverbs. Attributive adverbs such as *terribly, barely, hardest, luckily* make aspects of her thought process apparent and do so in no uncertain terms. By paying attention to the attributive adverbs that Sena employs, we begin to understand the personal significance of her trip through the tunnel. She employs attributive adverbs to qualify her psychological state by telling the reader that she *totally* "snapped." When she describes the difficulty of passing through the narrow tunnel, an effort that she *barely* weathered because the tunnel was *terribly* stuffy, we are not left unsure about Sena's feelings or the reasons for such feelings. Her use of attributive adverbs quite literally tells us that the *hardest* thing about the trip—which took about 30 minutes—was that she had to walk *stooped.*

As Daiute and Nelson (1997) point out, evaluation serves as a tool for young people as they situate themselves in their society. Magnified by her description of the trip through the tunnel, Sena's highly evaluative narrative reflects the unexpected and turbulent nature of her wartime society. Such activities involving heightened danger—across novel and precarious spaces—are described with greater semantic specificity than high-frequency, everyday activities, analogous to how the meaning of words becomes bleached and less salient through frequent exposure. The abrupt spatial changes Sena has lived through appear to have contributed to the development of a highly specific pattern of narrative evaluation. Because evaluation functions in the narrative to establish a point of personal interest and serve the developing awareness of self in relationship to the context (Daiute & Nelson, 1997), we interpret the overt and increased surfacing of evaluation as an intensified attempt to create a meaningful link between the self and the context of the activity.

Discussion: Significance of Evaluation when Narrating Extraordinary Circumstances

Analyzing adverbs in narratives that emerge from a "minor" regional crisis roughly 30 years ago amid the current "major" global crisis caused by the outbreak of the COVID-19 might strike some readers as a trivial pursuit. While narratives examined in this article came into existence as a response to a specific period of the Bosnian War, our work is not intended as solely a historical examination. Instead, we see these analyses as a prism, or tool, that grants us some distance and perspective necessary to make sense of what is happening to us and around us today. Conditions of radical change such as war, forced migrations, health crises, and environmental disasters that affects our experience of space and time are proliferating throughout our contemporary societies. As the world gradually learns to grapple with the effects of the coronavirus pandemic, the Russian Army is laying siege to Mariupol and other Ukrainian cities, amplifying the need to understand our contemporary world as permeated by the conditions of radical change. The question of how we understand a crisis at the time it is happening will determine how we respond to it. Hence, this work attempts to learn from the past to plan and prepare for the future.

Hence, the stakes of our project are high. As Freud (1920) teaches us, the less we objectively know about past responses to challenging situations, the more insecure and muddled our future responses will be. Recognizing that trauma is not the only or the natural response to a crisis is important. But equally as important is to understand that, following a period of radical change, we should not expect a brisk and straightforward return to the state of normalcy for most people. During prolonged, radical social change, the way people relate to their context changes. As our analyses show, a unique cultural context rendered in specific ways by the military siege continues to mediate the thought processes of our participants long after the acute period of crisis has passed.

In the previous sections, we offered a narrative analysis that illustrates the complex relationship of psychological processes to situated activities within physical spaces that engender them through narratives written by young

people. Not focusing on reified outcomes can yield insightful and important interpretations of experience in the aftermath of the crisis. We know that
spatial relations, both those lived and those contemplated, affect our conceptual structures and that the spatial terms may also affect our symbolic
representations of space. We have seen that extraordinary circumstances—
made manifest via the tunnel narrations—have led to more evaluative
descriptions. The evaluative nature of the tunnel narratives bears a resem-
blance to observations done on the language used under other challenging
circumstances. Such contexts may engage particular, sometimes peripheral
components of a person's communicative repertoire and can become unexpected, vital sources for coping and making sense of experience (Busch &
McNamara, 2020). Similarly, such narratives may range from detached to
relevant to— in our case—vivid and fully contextualized narratives that involve strong personal and emotional involvement and stance-taking.

The use of lexical items (such as evaluative words) in the text has been
approached from several angles, including age, style, and cognitive processing load. Our analysis—related to cognition and adverbial expressions
in narrations about conditions of radical change—provides a different perspective. We have shown that in new, unusual, and highly dangerous activities within unfamiliar spaces—such as the trip through the Sarajevo War
Tunnel—the sense-making processes of young people went into high gear.
The process becomes more evaluative, serving to develop an awareness of
the relationship between the self and the context. Bewildered by the setting
in which they were thrust, confused by how the activities are performed, and
unable to tell what is going on or know what to expect next, participants employ attributive adverbs to clarify and specify their impressions, feelings, and
thoughts and thereby understand the relationship between the self and the
space experienced.

References

Attanayake, V., McKay, R., Jeffres, M., Singh, S., Burkle, F., Jr., & Mills, E. (2009).
    Prevalence of mental disorders among children exposed to war: A systematic review of
    7,920 children. *Medicine, Conflict and Survival*, 25, 4–19.
Bassiouni, C. (1994 May 27). Final report of the United Nations Commission of Experts
    established pursuant to security council resolution 780. United Nations. Archived from
    the original on February 22, 2001.
Bruner, J. S., & Haste, H. (1987). Introduction. In J. S. Bruner & H. Haste (Eds.), *Making
    sense: The child's construction of the world* (pp. 1–25). Methuen.

Bonanno, G. A. (2004). Loss, trauma, and human resilience. *American Psychologist,* *59,* 20–28.

Busch, B., & McNamara, T. (2020). Language and trauma. An introduction. *Applied* *Linguistics, 41*(3), 323–333.

Clark, C. (2014). *The sleepwalkers: How Europe went to war in 1914.* Harper Perennial.

Cole, M. (1996). *Cultural psychology: A once and future discipline.* Harvard University Press.

Daiute, C. (2010). *Human development and political violence.* Cambridge University Press.

Daiute, C., & Lucić, L. (2010). Situated cultural development among youth separated by war. *International Journal of Intercultural Relations, 34,* 615–628.

Daiute, C., & Nelson, K. (1997). Making sense of the sense-making function of narrative evaluation. *Journal of Narrative and Life History, 7*(1-4), 207–215.

Fazel, M., Wheeler, J., & Danesh, J. (2005). Prevalence of serious mental disorder in 7000 refugees resettled in western countries: A systematic review. *Lancet, 365,* 1309–1314.

Freud, S. (1920). *A general introduction to psychoanalysis.* Horace Liveright.

Jahić, Dž., Halilović, S., & Palić, I. (2000). *Gramatika bosanskoga jezika.* Dom Štampe.

Labov, W., & Waletzky, J. (1967). Narrative analysis: Oral versions of personal experience. In J. Helm (Ed.), *Essays on the verbal and visual arts* (pp. 12–44). University of Washington Press.

Laor, N., Wolmer, L., Mayes, L. C., Golomb, A., Silverberg, D. S., Weizman, R., & Cohen, D. J. (1996). Israeli preschoolers under scud missile attacks: A developmental perspective on risk-modifying factors. *Archives of General Psychiatry, 53,* 416–423.

Lucić, L. (2013). Use of evaluative devices by youth for sense-making of culturally diverse interactions. *International Journal of Intercultural Relations, 37*(4), 434–449.

Lucić, L. (2016). Developmental affordances of war-torn landscapes: Growing up in Sarajevo under siege. *Human Development, 59,* 81–106.

Lucić, L. (2021). War Schools: Teaching innovations implemented across makeshift educational spaces during the military siege of Sarajevo. *Pedagogy, Culture & Society, 29*(4), 573–592.

Lucić, L., & Bridges, E. (2018). Ecological landscape in narrative thought: How siege survivors employ prepositions to make sense of war-torn Sarajevo. *Narrative Inquiry, 28*(2), 346–372.

Luria, A. R. (1976). *The cognitive development: Its cultural and social foundations.* Harvard University Press.

Maček, I. (2009). *Sarajevo under siege: Anthropology in wartime.* University of Pennsylvania Press.

Nelson, K. (1985). *Making sense: The acquisition of shared meaning.* Academic Press.

Nelson, K. (1996). *Language in cognitive development: The emergence of the mediated mind.* Cambridge University Press.

Ornstein, N., Miller, B. F., & Patel, K. (2020). The coming mental-health crisis. The Atlantic. MAY 14, 2020 https://www.theatlantic.com/ideas/archive/2020/05/coming-mental-health-crisis/611635/

Peltonen, K., & Punamäki, R. L. (2010). Preventive interventions among children exposed to trauma of armed conflict: A literature review. *Aggressive Behavior, 36*(2), 95–116.

Peterson, C., & McCabe, A. (1983). *Developmental psycholinguistics: Three ways of looking at a child's narrative.* Plenum Press.

Pilav, A. (2012). Before the war, war, after the war: Urban imageries for urban resilience. *International Journal of Disaster Risk Science, 3*(1), 23–37.

Pilav, A. (2020). Architects in war: Wartime destruction and architectural practice during the siege of Sarajevo. *Journal of Architecture, 25*, 697–716.

Ramscar, M., Matlock, T., & Boroditsky, L. (2010). Time, motion, and meaning: The experiential basis of abstract thought. In K. Mix, L. Smith & M. Gasser (Eds.), *The spatial foundations of language and cognition* (pp. 67–82). Oxford University Press.

Robinson, E., Sutin, A. R., Daly, M., & Jones, A. (2022). A systematic review and meta-analysis of longitudinal cohort studies comparing mental health before versus during the COVID-19 pandemic. *Journal of Affective Disorders, 296*, 567–576.

Rogoff, B. (2003). *The cultural nature of human development.* Oxford University Press.

Thabet, A. A., Abed, Y. & Vostanis, P. (2002). Emotional problems in Palestinian children living in a war zone: A cross-sectional study. *Lancet, 359*, 1801–1804.

Schwalm, D. E. (1985). Degree of difficulty in basic writing courses: Insights from the oral proficiency interview testing program. *College English, 47*(6), 629–640.

Solomon A. (2020). *When the pandemic leaves us alone, anxious and depressed.* New York Times. April 9, 2020 https://www.nytimes.com/2020/04/09/opinion/sunday/coronavirus-depression-anxiety.html

Vygotsky, L. S. (1934/1962). *Thought and language.* MIT Press.

Woodward, S. (1995). *Balkan tragedy: Chaos and dissolution after the Cold War.* Brookings Institution.

Zittoun, T. (2006). *Transitions: Development through symbolic resources.* Information Age.

PART II
THE SELF IN CRISIS

7

Plotless Stories and Unthought Knowns

Aspects of Psychological Life with COVID-19

Ruthellen Josselson

This chapter represents a talk written in May 2020, at what we now understand was the early stage of the pandemic when the quarantining and
lockdowns had lasted about six weeks in the eastern United States and the
US death toll was approaching 100,000. It was a time when, communally,
we were in shock from the changes in our lives and could not envision what
was ahead. The talk was an effort to give shape to and reflect on the storm
on the horizon. Images convey some of the affective experiences that cannot
be captured in words. As this chapter was written, 11 months later, despite
wrenching political events and the advent of vaccines, the psychological situation was still much the same, filled with uncertainty and vulnerability, plotless stories and unthought knowns. This chapter, then, attempts to describe
and analyze the particular kind of psychological vulnerability experienced in
response to the advent of the pandemic.

When I was asked to take part in a conference in May 2020, I was excited
about the possibility of talking to other scholars about the current situation
created by the pandemic. But when I considered what to talk about, I realized
that I had no data and therefore could not know anything in my usual ways,
which involve interviewing people in depth around a research question. And
then I realized that the whole question of knowledge is what is put at issue in
these surreal times. What can we know, and how do we know it?

Here is how the pandemic felt at its outset (Figure 7.1).

Here is what it looked like in the middle of March (Figure 7.2).

As one person said, "It's a weird feeling to miss the place where you are."

How do we make psychological sense of these images? What do they
mean to us on an individual level? My interest is in narrating—and
conceptualizing—the *subjective* experience of this pandemic and the ensuing
lockdown.

Ruthellen Josselson, *Plotless Stories and Unthought Knowns* In: *Narrative in Crisis*. Edited by: Martin Dege and Irene
Strasser, Oxford University Press. © Oxford University Press 2024. DOI: 10.1093/oso/9780197751756.003.0007

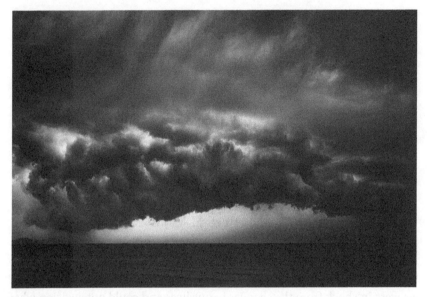

Figure 7.1 Storm clouds; dark and dramatic stormy clouds over sea.
Source: Adobe Stock.

I began then to think through various psychological theories to see if they provided frameworks or concepts with which to make sense of what is occurring in these surreal days and also to think about what would constitute data under these circumstances.

"Data" would imply some kind of narrative about what people have been experiencing and what meanings they make of their experiences. One way in which we think about narratives is that they are means of describing and linking events. Jerome Bruner, one of the great scholars of narratives, tells us that there is no narrative until there is a violation of the canonical (1990). What does he mean by this?

Culture provides an interpretive system for interdependent communal life. Culture provides us with a baseline of stories against which other narratives are juxtaposed. Taken-for-granted, invisible narratives receive no recognition and are not deemed worth telling. They operate "in the background," so to speak, the ordinary expectable events that fill our lives and we are unlikely to relate to others. Bruner refers to these narratives as *canonical*. People engage in active narrative construction only when these implicit narratives are "violated." We make meaning only out of those events that stand outside of the canonical narratives, for the canonical narratives are taken for granted,

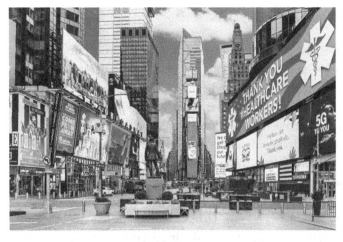

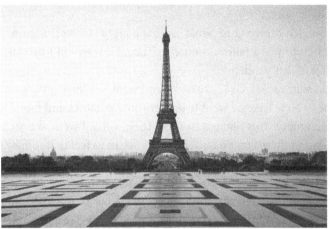

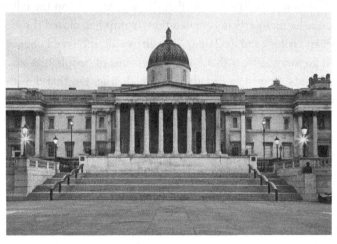

Figure 7.2 (a) Times Square and the empty streets of New York City, early spring 2020, during Coronavirus quarantine. (b) Eiffel Tower and the empty Trocadero, on a clear summer morning in Paris in 2020. (c) London's National Gallery building in the early morning, 2020.

Source: Adobe Stock.

they are already "understood" and thus need no meaning-making. Stories, on the other hand, make deviations from the canonical understandable. They take the form of describing a setting as well as an agent who performs some action toward a goal. A story has a plot linking events. When we don't see this link when someone tells us a story, we may ask them, "So what's your point?"

Canonical narratives vary by culture. What is unremarkable in one culture may seem quite outside the norm in another.

These are times where nearly everything is in violation of canonical narratives—in every culture. In every culture, people are experiencing the reality that life as we have known it has simply come to a stop. We have all never lived through such times before. Making meaning of these experiences, however, is challenging.

So how to understand what is happening to us? I turn now to autoethnography as a fallback source of data. How would I narrate my own experience of this pandemic?

I would start on March 12, 2020, when I went to a large grocery store near my home in New Jersey. I went to gather some potatoes and found the large potato bin empty. This seemed strange. Then, when I went to procure some butter, I found there was no butter. Then I began to feel that something very strange was going on. No potatoes, no butter. I asked one of the clerks who looked at me somewhat stupefied and said "Yes, and there is also no chicken, no toilet paper." In fact, the store was cleaned out of a lot of things. I was aware of the coronavirus at that point, but it felt to me like it was in China and in Italy. The *New York Times* from that day was focused on the falling stock market and the main article revealed that Trump had closed the US border to European visitors and declared, "The virus will not have a chance against us. It will go away." Places that had large groups of people like schools and sporting events, as well as Broadway, were closing. On that day, the *Times* reported, the virus was in 100 countries, had infected 120,000 people, and killed more than 4,300 around the world. Buried in that article, the *Times* also said, "Ordinary life in many places will no longer be the same for the foreseeable future as society adjusts to a new reality that transforms everything including the global economy and everyday social interactions—not just in far-off places on newscasts, but in the community right at home" (Baker, March 2020).

On my way home, I found potatoes and butter at another store and still could not begin to imagine what we were headed for. Indeed, my story of the potatoes and butter was not just a trivial noncanonical narrative. As a violation of my taken-for-granted assumptions, it was a piece of a shattering of canonical narratives everywhere.

Like many people I know, I tried to write a diary during this time, trying to keep track of experiences. But, like my friends, I found it impossible to find things to write about in the diary. "It was another day"—like all the other days. Circulating on social media was a meme that said, "Until further notice the days of the week are now called thisday, thatday, otherday, someday, yesterday, today and nextday!" What has been limited in our narrative capacity is both futurity and with it, intentionality. This is what creates the plotlessness.

My work life is unchanged from pre-virus times because I have for years been doing my work with my students, patients, and supervisees on the internet. I am not alone because my husband is with me and we have developed a kind of new routine. We work all day, take a walk, have dinner, then watch some engaging TV series and enjoy the sense of escape into some other reality. Then reading time—and I spend an inordinate amount of time reading news about the virus—then bed—and the next day, start again. What is most lost is planning—trips, excursions to theater or museums, visits with friends and family. As far as we can see, all our days will be the same, punctuated by grocery deliveries and Zoom social life. And even with those we love most, there is less and less to talk about—we are all in the "just another day" experience. Time itself has changed. Did we see the dolphins in the sea yesterday or last week? When did we last talk to your sister? Was the big storm two weeks ago or two months ago? Time is passing without markers.

I understand that universities, archives, and historical societies are rushing to collect and curate the personal accounts of how ordinary people are experiencing this sprawling public health crisis, but what I can see from the early submissions are plotless descriptions of emotions—fear, sadness, anger, and restlessness as well as moments of joy and hope. "Here's what I cooked" substitutes for often nameless emotions. Futurity, the setting of goals in time, has been compromised if not obliterated. Intentionality, the field of what one might do in a locked-down state, is severely limited. When the future is amorphous, the capacity to experience the present in narrative form changes.

Unlike other shared social catastrophes, such as natural events or human-caused destruction such as bombings, in which unaffected people either get on with their lives or go to help those who have been affected, this pandemic locks people into isolated spaces in fear. Regular life is suspended. It is too dangerous to go to help—at least in most cases. We are on pause—for an in-definite amount of time.

What then might be a collective narrative of these times? Looking at what the media is publishing, we seem to be amassing stories about loss, trauma, and challenge. Millions of people have endured heart-breaking losses from this virus—losses of loved ones, often under horrific circumstances where they were barred from saying goodbye to parents or spouses dying in care homes. Otherwise healthy loved ones have suddenly sickened and died, often denied medical attention that might have saved them. Each of the mourners has a painful narrative. Yet such narratives of loss are part of the canon of stories that accompany disasters that we are familiar with after such tragedies as 9/11, Hurricane Katrina, or the Japanese tsunami.

There are also growing numbers of loss narratives centering on unemploy-ment or business failures. Workers suddenly find themselves without income, dependent on unpredictable governmental benefits which they may or may not be eligible for and may or not be able to procure. People with successful businesses or occupations have found themselves suddenly facing financial ruin—and these, too, are tragic stories, but stories we have encountered be-fore in times of economic downturns or natural disasters, though none has been as widespread or deep as this one.

As I said before, I cannot speak directly from data and, in my isolated state, only have access to experiences of people like me who are among the privileged. We are privileged in that we have comfortable places to live and sufficient means to have food and the necessities of life. And yet there are profound psychological losses.

What is different about this pandemic are the often untold stories of losses, untold because they seem trivial in the face of others' tragic losses, but they involve loss of aspects of life and identity that are nevertheless highly dis-ruptive. Private disruptions involve the losses of expectable aspects of life, of routines that are foundational to our sense of ourselves, and these have psychological consequences that we are just beginning to try to understand. "Everyone is fine and adapting," a friend tells me, somewhat sheepishly, "but I can't play golf." This is a friend whose social life and sense of himself have long been organized about his golf game. For him, being kept from the golf course indefinitely is an enormous personal loss, and he is at pains to know what to do with himself without his golf game. And then there are the high school graduates who will not have a prom or a commencement ceremony, who don't know if universities they planned to attend will open in the fall.

And the college graduates who might have been seeking to begin their careers who now see no clear paths to doing so. In the face of death and bankruptcies, these seem minor, but they have deep psychological consequences.

Loss of a golf course or a prom is something people can eventually come to terms with, but they signify the loss of identity and a predictable world. Our psychological stability is based on feeling grounded, feeling that we can move through the world with some sense that we can take for granted certain cultural givens, like butter in the grocery store or a commencement when we graduate from high school or college. If these disappear, what can we count on?

The loss of grounding is central to trauma (see figure 7.3, Person in Sky in the Style of Dali). Traumatic events shatter one's sense of security,

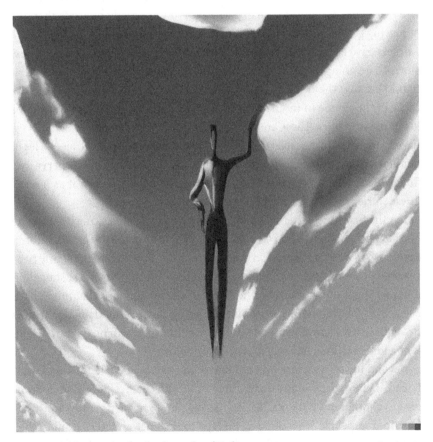

Figure 7.3 Person in sky, in the style of Dali.
Source: Created with the use of DALL-E, May 30, 2023.

making us feel helpless in a dangerous world. I strongly dislike using the word "trauma" loosely. The word "trauma" in this pandemic fits the experience of some first-responders and the healthcare workers trying to give medical assistance to an overload of people, too many to attend to, making life-and-death decisions when supplies and time are inadequate, risking their own and their family's lives to help others in the absence of enough personal protective equipment.

Traumatic experiences often involve a threat to life or safety, but any situation that leaves people feeling overwhelmed and isolated can result in trauma. And feelings of loss of self, brought on by losses in the cultural rituals that structure our lives, can involve psychological states akin to trauma. We cannot judge the extent of others' sense of loss and fear. It's not the objective circumstances that determine whether an event is traumatic, but the subjective emotional reaction to the experience. I am not ready to argue that loss of playing golf or going to a prom is a trauma on the level of what healthcare workers have endured, but I do think that these stories, which I call "plotless stories," are going to be part of our collective narrative of these times, often untold because they aren't stories in the usual sense and are often untold because of the shame in mourning the quotidian when others are grieving for losses of loved ones. These are stories about the tears in the fabric of life as we have known it, and, because they do not follow any of the usual trajectories of familiar stories, they are suppressed even while their effects can be pervasive. The overall shape of these stories is "The world/my world is not as it was." These stories refract, at a deeper level, our vulnerability.

For the first time in her life, my daughter is inaccessible to me because the border between the US and Canada is closed. I cannot see my grandchildren except on a screen. I long to feel them in my arms. I try to remember my two-year-old granddaughter with her soft little arms around my neck, snuggling into me. She is doing fine, but I have lost all those moments that might have been. And I have lost the possibility of going to help my daughter who is struggling to be a professor and take care of little ones with no daycare. There is no plot here, just a litany of loss of expectable life.

Beyond my own experience and that of my family and friends—and what I read in newspapers and magazines—the only data I have comes from my psychotherapy patients. All of the people I see for therapy are high-functioning people who came to therapy to deal with relatively mild states of anxiety or depression or difficulties in their relationships. My friends say to me, "I guess you are hearing a lot about anxiety and depression brought on from the COVID-19 situation from your patients." But the reality is that I am not. With most of my patients, people who live all over the world, we now check in about "how things are" in our home places and recognize that, with some minor variations in lockdowns and reopenings, we are all pretty much confined to our private spaces. Then we go on to the meat of therapy, which is dealing with the selves that they have been and are trying to better understand and change. The underlying assumption—which I find myself sharing—is that we will one day go back to "normal" and be who we have always been in a world that is as it has always been.

That is, perhaps, the central arc of the larger plot of the pandemic story, a plot we are collectively developing. There is a before and there will be an after while the present is a time in limbo, a waystation between the self in a world we have known and the self in a world that we will find ourselves in when this pandemic "goes away."

This brings me to the concept of the "unthought known." The idea was developed by psychoanalyst Christopher Bollas (1987) to represent what we know through sensory or preconscious experience but are not able to think about. It is a hallmark of infants' earliest experience of being, feeling themselves in a particular kind of embrace by those who form their world. These sensory experiences form the basic structure of the personality, but they are felt rather than thought. In later life, unthought knowns are things we may have forgotten or find ourselves playing out in action. We may have an intuitive sense for these early experiences but cannot yet put them into words and cannot direct our thinking toward them. In the past several years, there has been an upsurge of ideas about this implicit dimension of experience—that which is in some sense known but not yet available to thought or language. Some have termed this "unformulated experience," and psychoanalysis is paying more attention to these states of being. The unthought known is something that is there and not there, "more than can be put into words." It can be communicated in image and perhaps in metaphor. And poets such as T. S. Eliot have tried to capture it.

> We shall not cease from exploration
> And the end of all our exploring
> Will be to arrive where we started
> And know the place for the first time.
> Through the unknown, remembered gate
> When the last of earth left to discover

Is that which was the beginning;
At the source of the longest river
The voice of the hidden waterfall
And the children in the apple-tree
Not known, because not looked for
But heard, half-heard, in the stillness
Between two waves of the sea.

— T.S. Eliot, Excerpt of poem "Four Quartets"

Wilfred Bion (1994) was working with similar ideas when he wrote about the distinction between beta and alpha function. *Beta elements* are most evident in the infant who is filled with sensory experience that they cannot think about. Beta elements are felt but not represented in thought, which would be *alpha function*. In human development, it is the mother's thinking capacity, what Bion called alpha function, which contains the beta elements, the sensory experience of her child, and this, over time, makes it possible for the child to become able to think. Alpha function transforms the undigested facts of internal and external experience into thought. We can think of this as the difference between apprehending something and comprehending it.

One unthought known—the beta elements—in the current crisis is what Ernest Becker (1973) called "the rumble of panic underneath everything (p. 284)." We have a heightened awareness of the existential contradiction between having a symbolic self that seems to give humans infinite worth in a timeless scheme of things and our physical selves, which involve a mortal body. To Becker, culture is part of an immortality project of a symbolic self that serves the denial of death. As the coronavirus is a mortal danger to our physical selves, we see how the adjustments to flee it have threatened what we know of culture. As we withdraw from one another in fear, economic and social arrangements are in disarray and cultural supports seem to be either disappearing or on hold for some unspecified amount of time (See Figure 7.4 for Munch's depiction of this emotional state).

Unformulated experience is a moment-to-moment state of vagueness and possibility. These beta experiences—the realm of the unthought known— form the painful and disruptive sense that the normal is gone and we cannot yet think about what might take its place. I am struck by how frequently, when I talk to friends, they say, "I can't think about that." Or, "I don't want to think about that." These phrases come up when our conversation drifts to the future. In the current situation, we have lost our ability to plan and, with it,

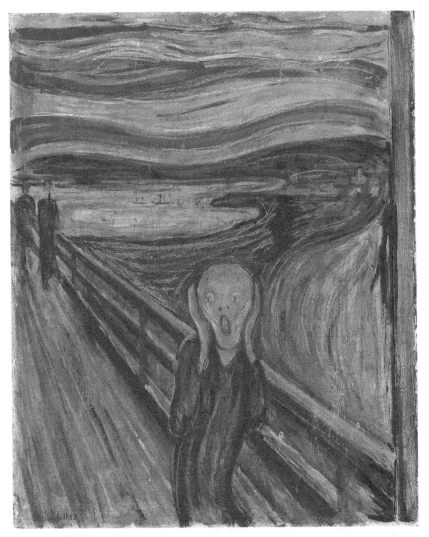

Figure 7.4 "The Scream" by Edvard Munch, Munch Museum, Oslo.
Source: Public Domain.

the capacity to envision the future. The future itself has become an unthought known and to think about that is terrifying. In early life, beta experiences are transformed by a container, someone whose thinking enables our own capacity to think. In Bion's formulation, that is the function of the mother. In order to think about the future in the current crisis, we would need a container, someone who has a capacity to think about it in much the way the mother can soothe the infant through her capacity to think. Is there anyone or anything that can offer the alpha function that we need, the reassurance that it will all turn out okay because they are thinking for us? Can anyone hold for us the promise that we can return to some semblance of life as we've known it?

Unthought knowns can be collective as well as individual. We each have our private demons and apocalyptic worries, but these can exist at the larger levels of society as well. What are we, as a collective, keeping at bay, keeping ourselves from thinking about?

To think about the future, we need knowledge of the present and this, too, is obscure. Right now, our knowledge of reality is mediated through screens and print media. From our locked-down state, we rely on others to tell us what is going on in the world even as we recognize that everyone has only a very limited view. This, in part, accounts for the inordinate amount of time I spend reading news—trying to get a sense of knowing something about what the world is like and that others know something about it. The *New York Times* has become my, however imperfect, container.

If we look back on the first month of the pandemic, we note that the genome of the novel coronavirus, now named COVID-19, was sequenced in China within a couple of days. This was something of a miracle of modern technology. Our science reacted quickly, and we could identify the foe. Yet, since then, our capacity to know has faltered or ground to a halt. We still know little about the transmissibility of this virus, which leaves us not knowing just where to identify risk. As a result, we are, in effect, directed to be afraid of nearly everything—all other people who we don't live with, all surfaces outside our private spaces.

We look to our leaders for containment, much as we once, as children, looked to our parents. Surely someone must know what to do; the scientists can find a way to stop this monstrous thing before it kills us all. Leaders are charged with the responsibility of looking out for our welfare: Surely, they will find a way for us to live safely while the scientists find the solution. But, as we have seen, except in a few fortunate countries where leadership has been efficient, timely, and wise, our leaders have been focused on their own political advantage and are willing to lie and dissemble in order to create a self-serving narrative. Conspiracy theories with their alternative narratives are proliferating. Collectively we engage in painful epistemic disputes with detailed and often threatening counterrealities. But we need some form of shared reality in order to be able to think. It is thinking that wards off panic and containment that makes it possible for the alpha function of thought. One of the most present dangers is losing our collective capacity to think at all.

This experience has taught me much about the containment function of leadership. One leader who embodied containment for me is Andrew Cuomo, who, in his daily briefings, sifted through available information, marked problems, offered good sense, and honestly told us what he didn't know. He enacted a thinking man—someone taking the elements of what we know and assembling them into some kind of rational whole, all the while indicating that he was as frightened and sad as we were. He didn't offer panaceas or solutions. Rather, with his graphs and charts, he demonstrated thinking. On the day I was initially writing this in early May 2020, someone asked Governor Cuomo when he thought New York would reopen, and he said he didn't know. I was struck by how containing this admission was. If someone had asked Trump the same question, he would have offered an arbitrary date. But Cuomo seemed, at some level, to understand how not knowing was highly containing. It meant that someone with the amount of authority that he possessed would be thinking about it and delaying making a decision until he had some degree of certainty that reopening made sense. He was implicitly inviting us to allow him to do some thinking for us, to assemble all those bits of terrible stories we were reading and hearing about into something like a coherent narrative that could lead to an imagined future.

So, we have been living now in limbo in a world beyond our understanding, a world filled with fear of the invisible in which we are locking ourselves in order to keep safe. Even for people in places where there have been few cases of COVID-19, there is fear of the unseen—the invisible enemy could still appear and strike as it has in other places. Even those far away from epicenters are bombarded with images of people dying with relative suddenness and often in terrible circumstances. I doubt that there is anyone on the planet that the rumble of panic has not touched.

We turn to history as a container as well. We have been here before. But it is interesting how our collective history has banished prior pandemics to the realm of the unthought known. Just a few decades after the 1918 Spanish flu pandemic, which killed more people than World War I, the most important American history textbooks by the distinguished likes of Arthur M. Schlesinger Jr., Richard Hofstadter, Henry Steele Commager, and Samuel Eliot Morison said not a word about it. It is similarly missing from Yuval Harari's sweeping account of human history in *Sapiens*. History, evidently, is a record of human intentionality. We want to assume that our human species controls its own destiny. We're in charge! we think. Like historians, we cannot accept that brainless packets of RNA and DNA can capsize the human enterprise in a few weeks or months. In the early part of the 20th century, the flu was incomprehensible. The influenza virus wasn't even identified until 1931. Now we know what the COVID-19 virus is but, so far, that hasn't done us a lot of good. So, the sense of helplessness and impending disaster continue to lurk in the unthought known.

Beyond the losses of life, our economic order has been dismantled, and we are told to expect worldwide economic depression. The panicky thought here is, "Will we have the food and other resources to sustain us? Will we be able to maintain the social order, or is anarchy on the horizon?" These are questions that lurk as unthinkable but vaguely foreboding.

But there are others who are taking the unknown future in a different way. Can we use the devastation to build a better world? Can we see this pandemic as a preview of climate change, which would be a lot worse in terms of destruction and dislocation of the world as we know it? Could we take this more seriously now as a collective and work to prevent it? Can we restore our human intentionality to a world in which we have thus far been rendered rather helpless?

And what of our economic structures? We have been rethinking what it means to be an "essential" worker. These are the service workers who cannot work from home because their physical presence in getting food from the fields to our tables is absolutely necessary—from those who are picking our vegetables to those who are stocking shelves in grocery stores to those who are driving the vehicles to bring them to our doors. Yet these "essential" workers are the lowest paid in our economic system. Is this how we want to proceed in the future? Do we now understand better how income inequality and limited access to healthcare also imply vulnerability for the rich who rely on workers to make the products that create their wealth? Is this how we want things to be going forward? The future doesn't have to be bleak. If every crisis is an opportunity, we can also work with the crystals of hope—hopes for transformation for the better can also be part of the unthought known.

So, what will be the shape of the collective ending to the COVID-19 story once we create a plot for it? Will it be . . . and then we all went back to normal? Or . . . and then we tried to build a better world? Can it end with a new day dawning?

And on a more personal level, we may ask ourselves, do we really *want* the ending to be "and then I went back to life as it was" (unlikely in any case) or, "I have a new recognition of our social interdependence and will modify my life to respect it better."

We can be certain that this experience is changing us in ways we cannot yet see—in that sense, a part of the as-yet unthought unknown. How our personal and collective stories will be emplotted, as they eventually will, is still unknown. We are still in limbo, caught in a surreal present headed for an even more uncertain future. Let us hope for the best.

References

Baker, P. (2020, March 11). U.S. to suspend most travel from europe as world scrambles to fight pandemic. https://www.nytimes.com/2020/03/11/us/politics/anthony-fauci-coronavirus.html

Becker, E. (1973). *The denial of death*. Simon and Schuster.

Bion, W. R. (1994). *Learning from experience*. Jason Aronson.

Bollas, C. (1987). *The shadow of the object: Psychoanalysis of the unthought known*. Columbia University Press.

Bruner, J. (1990). *Acts of meaning*. Harvard University Press.

8

Coping Personally and Politically
with World Crises

Can It Be Done Wisely?

Michel Ferrari and Melanie Munroe

The current global COVID-19 crisis is unprecedented in many ways and yet "crisis," existing or potential, seems perennial to human life. Certainly, for years, we have been hearing of a "refugee crisis," the 2007–2008 financial crises, and the global climate crisis—itself often identified as a potential trigger for future global crises. On the social and cultural level, we have #MeToo, Black Lives Matter, global surveillance disclosures, and the Canadian residential schools crisis for Indigenous First Nations. And, of course, personal crises, in the form of physical or verbal abuse or an existential loss of meaning that can generate depression or anxiety.

In this chapter, we discuss the idea of wisdom as an aspect of posttraumatic growth, both personal and communal. In dealing with crises, such as the COVID-19 pandemic or the current conflict in Ukraine, personal resilience and communal coping can lead to increased growth at the individual and community levels. In particular, we explore the potential for coping wisely with crises to foster a more resilient post-crisis world.

Crisis

The *Oxford English Dictionary* (online) defines crisis as "a vitally important or decisive stage in the progress of something, a turning-point, or a state of affairs in which a decisive change for better or worse is imminent." Historically, this definition was applied to the course of disease and astrological influences on human destiny, but now it is often applied to times of political or economic difficulty, insecurity, and suspense.

Michel Ferrari and Melanie Munroe, *Coping Personally and Politically with World Crises* In: *Narrative in Crisis*. Edited by: Martin Dege and Irene Strasser, Oxford University Press. © Oxford University Press 2024. DOI: 10.1093/oso/9780197751756.003.0008

Personal Crisis: An Opportunity for Individual
Posttraumatic Growth

In *Twilight of the Idols*, Nietzsche (1889/1998) famously wrote, "Aus der Kriegsschule des Lebens. — Was mich nicht umbringt, macht mich starker" [Out of the war-school of life, What doesn't kill me makes me stronger], and, indeed, many people who have had traumatic experiences claim to have grown from them—often, they say they have gained wisdom through coping with adversity.

Inspired by Janoff-Bulman's (1992, 2004) work, Tedeschi, Calhoun, and colleagues (1996, 2004; Blevins & Tedeschi, 2022; Calhoun et al., 2010) were the first to systematically study this experience, which they called "posttraumatic growth." They found that through iterative reappraisal, set-shifting, and decentering, people often report that their understanding of their own role in an experienced crisis becomes better articulated, more satisfying and more meaningful. Over the long term, people do not return to where they began before the crisis. Posttraumatic growth is expressed in five main ways: (1) an increased appreciation for life in general, (2) more meaningful interpersonal relationships, (3) an increased sense of personal strength, (4) changed priorities, and (5) a richer existential and spiritual life.

Although Nietzsche's dictum is not true for everyone, approximately 70% of trauma survivors report experiencing positive change in at least one life domain (Linley & Joseph, 2004). These rates are very high and—while they may in part reflect a desire to claim some positive benefit from difficult life experiences—they signify the importance of understanding how individuals can cope successfully with these types of events.

Tedeschi and Calhoun (2004) propose a model for understanding the process of posttraumatic growth that includes individual characteristics, support and disclosure, and, more centrally, significant cognitive processing involving cognitive structures threatened or nullified by the traumatic events. More specifically, they found a need to reimagine ourselves in ways that make us wiser. The development of posttraumatic growth is theorized to lead to a sense of wisdom about the world, and, potentially, over time, to greater satisfaction with life. Posttraumatic growth mutually interacts with life wisdom and the development of the life narrative; it is an ongoing process, not a static outcome.

In other words, how we cope with personal crisis is the key to developing wisdom and growing from adversity. According to Tedeschi and Calhoun's (2004) model, people first experience crisis as a *seismic disruption of core assumptions* about themselves and the world through events that are unusual, threatening, uncontrollable, and often irreversible. Tedeschi, Calhoun, and colleagues have studied a range of such seismic events at different social scales in a wide range of personal, social, and ecological contexts including a relationship ending, grief and bereavement, cancer, war, and natural disasters (see Blevins & Tedeschi, 2022).

Although natural (and even important to later recovery), one's immediate response is potentially debilitating distress that evokes forms of coping that at first may be instinctive and unpleasant (e.g., intrusive rumination on unwanted cognitive pattern, unwanted thoughts and images). Later, this coping can come to involve deliberative rumination that helps rebuild one's worldview from new core assumptions through a variety of broadly metacognitive transformational coping strategies that support resilient and positive reinterpretation of life events that make one stronger through having weathered adversity or help one abandon unobtainable goals. Ideally, such deliberate rumination is also supported socially: indeed, if the environment is safe for *verbal disclosure* to supportive others (Lindstrom et al., 2013) and *written disclosure,* one can find social support for both cognitive and emotional aspects of trauma processing. More broadly, societal master narratives influence how individuals process trauma and coping; for example, master narratives of redemption can give meaning to suffering and hope of a better future—albeit one that must be negotiated in light of one's intersectional personal identity (McLean & Syed, 2015; McLean, Pasupathi & Syed, 2023). Indeed, posttraumatic growth is inherently a redemptive narrative (Blevins & Tedeschi, 2022).

One example of a cultural narrative of redemption is that of Edmund Metatawabin, as portrayed in his book, *Up Ghost River* (2014). Edmund Metatawabin is a survivor of the residential school system in Canada who struggled with a dependency on alcohol during his early adulthood but found healing through culturally appropriate healthcare that emphasized Indigenous healing practices. Following this, he later became a community leader who convened the Keykaywin Conference, where 750 survivors recounted the abuse they experienced at the residential schools, leading to the arrest and sentencing of seven church staff and bringing some sense of resolution and justice to the survivors (Metatawabin, 2014). This activism continued through his involvement in the Indian Residential School Settlement Agreement and as a leader in the fight against the Canadian government to release confidential residential school documents (Metatawabin, 2014).

Posttraumatic growth is also evident in narratives from our recent studies of trauma survivors. For example, one participant detailed their experience in dealing with the aftermath of Hurricane Harvey that made landfall on Texas and Louisiana in August 2017. Initially, their family "lost everything" during the flood and the participant said that "it took us over a year to fully recover and left us in financial ruin." Although this event was extremely difficult for them, and they almost lost their lives, they were now able to reframe the event in a positive light in order to cope with what had happened, saying, "this event made me realize how fragile life and material things are. It made me appreciate life in a more deeper level while reminded me that nothing is eternal and we should be thankful for each moment we live." In other words, this survivor experienced meaning and redemption from their experience that allowed them to appreciate the fragility of life, clearly demonstrating an increased appreciation of life—one of Tedeschi and Calhoun's domains of potential posttraumatic growth.

Although Tedeschi and colleagues are careful to say that positive events can be equally self-transformative and that trauma is not necessary for posttraumatic growth, nevertheless, personal crises can be a catalyst toward fulfillment, growth, and wisdom by refining or acquiring cognitive and emotional resources that rebuild assumptions through a more sophisticated narrative about oneself and the world that ultimately restores one's life satisfaction—what Tedeschi and Calhoun associate with developing wisdom.

Meta-analysis shows that posttraumatic growth more strongly predicts better health outcomes when more time has elapsed since the trauma; individuals may be particularly likely to experience growth in areas that match their pre-trauma personality dispositions (Tennen & Affleck, 1998). For example, extraverts may become more socially sophisticated: cognitive complexity, self-efficacy, and dispositional hope may also help in aligning posttraumatic growth with resilience of other kinds. Indeed, optimism, extraversion, and openness to experience have been identified as significant predictors of increased levels of posttraumatic growth (Tedeschi & Calhoun, 1996).

A study by Frazier et al. (2009) shows that retrospective reports of growth, such as the Posttraumatic Growth Inventory, may measure something different from actual pre- to post-trauma change and may rather measure a type of "illusory growth" (Fleeson, 2014). And Yanez et al. (2011) found no relationship between prospective and retrospective measurements of posttraumatic growth. Most studies have utilized retrospective self-reports, which are imperfect assessments of veridical change in participants' lives (Jayawickreme et al., 2021). Methodological improvements to the study of individual posttraumatic growth are needed to confirm developmental trajectories of growth over time before and following a crisis or traumatic event.

Developing Wisdom from Crises

Defining Wisdom

As Arnold and Linden (2022) point out, "wisdom" is a complex multidimensional capacity/competence to address life's problems big and small—both on the landscape of action (doing well) and on that of conscious experience (feeling well) (Bruner, 1986). More specifically, wisdom is an expertise in living well (Baltes & Smith, 1990; Tsai, 2022) which is acquired by all people, in varying degrees, and used to solve not only crises but also everyday nuisances, if they are thought to ultimately relate to matters of ultimate importance in life.

Thus, wisdom is not about using a specific coping strategy, but about discerning the most appropriate ways of coping with a crisis—a meta-perspective that monitors the availability and appropriateness of different potential courses of action (Baltes & Staudinger, 2000) given knowledge about oneself and the situation (Ferrari & Munroe, 2022; Glück, 2022).

Put another way, wisdom as expertise in living well involves a complex set of skills and metaskills that make addressing an important problem more likely. Arnold and Linden (2022) identify four main wisdom dimensions that must be developed and coordinated: (1) one's view of the world— (factual, procedural, contextual) knowledge, value relativism; (2) one's view of others—perspective taking, empathy; (3) one's view of the Self—self-relativism' self-distancing, and aspirational relativism, including a metaview of own experience that perceives and accepts one's emotions; and, (4) one's view of the future—forgiveness and accepting the past, tolerating uncertainty, long-term perspective.

Wisdom is therefore both a continuously developing personal resource and a characteristic of a particular moment of one's life that allow for wisdom to further develop (Glück, 2022; Webster, 2022). These personal wisdom resources are best considered a self-organizing dynamic system that perceives situational possibilities, not a disjoined set of characteristics— an emergent expertise that (potentially) evolves through self-reflection and experience articulated in narratives about important experiences of coping with adversity, partially shaped by cultural master narratives and the powers and prejudices they imply (Glück, 2022; McLean, Pasupathi & Syed, 2023; Mansfield, 2022; Webster, 2022).

Acquiring the wisdom needed to cope wisely with crises and grow from them may require prerequisite resources, what Glück (2022) calls five "wisdom resources" of her MORE model. These resources are integral to how people appraise and deal with life challenges prospectively and learn from them retrospectively: (1) managing uncertainty and uncontrollability, (2) openness, (3) reflectivity, (4) emotional sensitivity, and (5) emotion regulation. They might be considered metaheuristics to gain the most from life situations.

According to Glück, these five MORE resources develop asynchronously, as follows:

1. Openness and 2. emotional sensitivity are present from infancy,
3. Reflectivity develops progressively, and not fully before adolescence,
4. Emotion regulation and 5. management of uncertainty and uncontrollability are outcomes of learning from life in themselves.

Self-compassion is another important resource that may only emerge along with self-conscious emotions like pride and shame (Bluth et al., 2022). Self-compassion may be a prerequisite to developing the MORE resources or deploying them. Self-compassion is also a metastrategy that supports taking other perspectives—a kind of relational meaning-meaning that promotes posttraumatic growth (Bluth et al., 2022)[1].

---

[1] The three aspects of self-compassion as defined by Bluth, following Neff (2003), are
  (1) mindfulness (related to openness),
  (2) common humanity (related to reflective, self-transcendence), and
  (3) self-kindness (an "emotional wisdom" [Germer & Siegel, 2012] or, perhaps better, a metaemotion).

As Ricoeur (1992; also Bruner, 1986) notes, narratives frame how the self is construed, with implications for well-being and coping with present and future adversity. Self-compassion informs a self-narrative frame that engages wisdom-related metacognitive knowledge, emotion, and desire through what Buber calls an 'I-thou' (rather than an 'I-it') relationship to oneself.

Of course, these resources are not just internal to the person but also present in their social context—like Ungar's (2012) ecological model of resilience and Grossmann's (2017) situated wise reasoning—and thus cultivated not only in social interactions, but also within historical communities in the face of adversity.

All this shows that posttraumatic growth must be understood within the context of a person's broader biographical development; that is, where a person finds themselves in their life when the trauma takes place—a biographical moment that extends beyond themselves to include their sociohistorical setting. Triggering events reflect personal meaning within one's own "biographicity" (Alheit, 1995) that are "self-shattering." Triggering or focal traumatic events can only be understood in light of their meaning or significance for the person at that biographical moment of their lives—not as an isolated occurrence, but within a larger narrative for and about the self and others in the world (Bruner, 1986; Ricoeur, 1992)—a point not fully developed by Tedeschi and colleagues.

This relates back to our ability to transcend the potentially traumatic COVID crisis that we are currently facing. Research from our lab has shown that the presence of meaning in life and self-transcendent wisdom had the strongest positive association with change in perceived well-being during the COVID-19 pandemic (Kim et al., 2021). Self-transcendent wisdom contributed to well-being over and above coping styles and predicted change in well-being for people using most coping styles (except those using religious coping) (Kim et al., 2021). Self-transcendent wisdom may be one of the biggest contributors to positive transformation, when an individual lacks adaptive coping strategies to deal with crises. Additionally, participants with high levels of self-transcendent wisdom reported being involved in more personal projects that deepened their connection with other people and their community (Kim et al., 2021).

Humanitarian Crisis: An Opportunity for Collective Posttraumatic Growth

Personal posttraumatic growth provides a template for collective posttraumatic growth. However, in this case, it is not individuals, but our collective life together as nations and as humanity that is reimagined. Narvarez (2014) suggests starting with parenting and education, since secure parenting creates conditions for coping and wisdom. However, for those not fortunate enough to be well-socialized, self-authorship is potentially available to all adults (Bauer, 2021). Likewise, for nations, such as Ukraine: calamities can teach us something about the kind of society we are and the kind of society we would like ourselves to become. But whether this is possible depends in part on political leadership and culture and entrenched interests. And that is what progressive voices need to advocate for wisely—a different image of wisdom more closely associated with rhetoric and civic duty, in addition to personal self-transcendence or reimagining (Edmondson, 2012).

Collective posttraumatic growth can be defined "as benefits perceived in the community and society in response to collective trauma experiences: Community learning reflected in collective emotions, emotional climate, beliefs, values and social behaviors" (Páez et al., 2013, p.18). Collective or community posttraumatic growth can increase resilience through a governmental response that provides individuals with economic resources, reduces inequity, and attends to the areas of greatest vulnerability (Norris et al., 2008). Communities must exercise flexibility and have effective communication when faced with uncertainty (Norris et al., 2008).

Collectively coping with crises requires collective coping strategies, such as instrumental support from friends or family, social sharing, and participating in rituals and/or spiritual practices (Rhodes & Tran, 2012). Some of the main features of communal coping involve a shared collective experience, shared appraisals (thinking and acting as if the stressor is "our problem"), social sharing, and mobilization of social relations (people need to share responsibilities and act together to face the crisis) (Lyons et al., 1998). This can be seen through the various social and community movements during the COVID-19 pandemic. For example, a movement on social media in Canada called #Caremongering consisted of Facebook groups that helped support vulnerable members of the community (Seow et al., 2021). Indeed, a sense of community is a protective factor for both well-being and for lessening the impact of COVID on life domains such as family relationships or mental health (Mannarini et al., 2021).

Different types of communal coping typically seen following disaster include: changing the situation and social relationships (active coping and social support), avoidance ("healthy denial"), redirecting attention (self-distraction) and cognitive change (positive reappraisal), and emotion regulation (self-control and expression) (see Wlodarczyk et al., 2016a). Things like "healthy denial" (Druss & Douglas, 1988) early on following a traumatic event may initially be beneficial, allowing individuals to control their processing of the event to avoid becoming overwhelmed (Butler et al., 2005; Tedeschi & Calhoun, 1995).

Communal coping aims to reduce the negative impact of traumatic experience, which can lead to posttraumatic growth and may subsequently increase well-being (Wlodarczyk et al., 2016b). Communal coping is also associated with lower levels of psychological distress (Koehly et al., 2008) and better recovery (Hobfoll et al., 2008) in the context of natural disasters and traumatic events that affect families and communities. The reconstruction of social relations, a sense of belonging, and a social identity based on values such as solidarity and community cohesion can help counter the effects of a crisis (Lykes et al., 2007). For example, posttraumatic growth after natural disasters appears to be higher in more collectivistic cultures compared to individualistic cultures (Wlodarczyk et al., 2016b). Moreover, increased identification with a communal group as a consequence of the collective experience can act to ameliorate some of the negative consequences of the adversity (Muldoon et al., 2017). Having a strong sense that the group can cope with the crisis leads to both more posttraumatic stress and posttraumatic growth, as these two concepts tend to co-occur (Muldoon et al., 2017). Having a stronger collective efficacy and community identity also are related to posttraumatic growth following a natural disaster (Muldoon et al., 2017). Posttraumatic growth in response to disaster is driven by beliefs in the strength of one's national and local communities in the face of a crisis (Muldoon et al., 2017).

Disaster Communication

One important aspect of communally or collectively coping wisely with crises is disaster communication. For example, during the crisis, it is important to connect with loved ones, correct inaccurate reports, and confirm information about the disaster (Spialek & Houston, 2018). Research across 58 countries at the beginning of the COVID-19 pandemic found that the more false information was spread over social media, such as information that would downplay COVID-19 or that would doubt the effectiveness of masks, the more the case count would increase (Kong et al., 2021). For example, Canada had lower social media use and less COVID-19 cases at the beginning of the pandemic in comparison to the United States (Kong et al., 2021). However, receiving instrumental or emotional support from loved ones (Spialek et al., 2019) and confirming information about what is happening during the event (Tian et al., 2016) has been connected with increased levels of posttraumatic growth. After the event, it is also important that disaster communication includes telling stories, assisting with recovery, and encouraging growth in others (Spialek & Houston, 2018). Sharing and telling stories is one aspect of interpersonal communication between individuals that can help promote broader posttraumatic growth following disaster (Tedeschi & Calhoun, 2004) within what Hayes (2010a, 2010b) calls the 'wisdom ecosystem' that includes communal meaning and dialogue.

Another important piece of disaster communication is the governmental response to the crisis. The quality of the government response can predict higher levels of growth or posttraumatic stress depending on whether it was interpreted as positive or negative following natural disasters. Indeed, if the quality of the response was interpreted as negative, problems may persist months later, with survivors wondering how things might have been different if there was a better governmental response (Rhodes & Tran, 2012). The feeling that we are being taken care of helps to promote a "healing community" in the face of crisis (Tyler & Rogers, 2005).

Four Layers of Support in Developing Wise Coping

Magid and Boothby (2013) describe how the 2007 Inter-Agency Standing Committee (IASC) *Guidelines on Mental Health and Psychosocial Support in Emergency Settings* use a social ecologic model to promote resilience that further articulates Hayes' (2010a, 2010b) wisdom ecosystem. Because most psychosocial support is provided from within a community and not by outside interveners, the IASC Guidelines propose programs that form a four-level pyramid. From the base of the pyramid to the top, these four levels are (1) basic services and security; (2) community and family supports; (3) focused, non-specialized, supports; and (4) specialized services. Each layer of the pyramid is essential and must be implemented simultaneously; however, the supports near the base of the pyramid tend to benefit the most people in a community, while the mental health style interventions at the top tend to benefit only a few individuals needing personally-targeted care. In our view, coping wisely with crises, personally and communally, should be designed to reduce risk and create opportunities for posttraumatic growth in wisdom at all four of these levels of the wisdom ecology.

Conclusion

In this chapter, we have tried to show how Nietzsche's famous dictum can be made a reality. Many people do grow from personal and communal crisis, however, doing so requires enacting Tedeschi and Calhoun's (1996, 2004) model at all four levels of the IASC pyramid in a way that necessarily relies on existing personal and ecological wisdom and wisdom resources—including self-compassion. In so doing, we go beyond an individual personal model of growth to address communal coping and collective posttraumatic growth, equally important to developing wisdom in response to crisis. Collectively we have more strength and more wisdom than any one of us alone, as we all have clearly seen during the COVID-19 pandemic.

References

Alheit, P. (1995). Biographical Learning. Theoretical Outline, Challenges and Contradictions of a New Approach in Adult Education. In P. Alheit, A. Bron-Wojciechowska, E. Brugger, & P. Dominicé (Eds.), *The Biographical Approach in European Adult Education* (pp. 57–74). Vienna: Verband Wiener Volksbildung.

Arnold, C., & Linden, M. (2022). Wisdom therapy in overcoming trauma and burdens of life. In M. Munroe & M. Ferrari (Eds.), *Post-traumatic growth to psychological well-being: Coping wisely with adversity (Lifelong learning book series, vol 30)* (pp. 207–219). Springer Cham.

Baltes, P. B., & Smith, J. (1990). The psychology of wisdom and its ontogenesis. In R. J. Sternberg (Ed.), *Wisdom: Its nature, origins, and development* (pp. 87–120). New York: Cambridge University Press.

Baltes, P. B., & Staudinger, U. M. (2000). A metaheuristic (pragmatic) to orchestrate mind and virtue toward excellence. *American Psychologist, 55,* 122–136.

Bauer, J. J. (2021). *The transformative self: Personal growth, narrative identity, and the good life.* New York: Oxford University.

Blevins, C. L., & Tedeschi, R. G. (2022). Posttraumatic growth & wisdom: Processes and clinical applications. In M. Munroe & M. Ferrari (Eds.), *Post-traumatic growth to psychological well-being: Coping wisely with adversity (Lifelong learning book series, vol 30)* (pp. 11–26). Springer Cham.

Bluth, K., Lathren, C., & Park, J. (2022). Self-compassion as a Protective Factor for Adolescents Experiencing Adversity. In M. Munroe & M. Ferrari (Eds.), *Post-traumatic growth to psychological well-being: Coping wisely with adversity (Lifelong learning book series, vol 30)* (pp. 111–126). Springer Cham.

Bruner, J. (1986). *Actual minds, possible worlds.* Harvard University Press.

Butler, L. D., Blasey, C. M., Garlan, R. W., McCaslin, S. E., Azarow, J., Chen, X. H., Desjardins, J. C., DiMiceli, S., Seagraves, D. A., Hastings, T. A., Kraemer, H. C., & Spiegel, D. (2005). Posttraumatic growth following the terrorist attacks of September 11, 2001: Cognitive, coping, and trauma symptom predictors in an internet convenience sample. *Traumatology, 11*(4), 247–267. https://doi.org/10.1177/15347656050 1100405

Calhoun, L. G., Cann, A., & Tedeschi, R. G. (2010). The posttraumatic growth model: Socio-cultural considerations. In T. Weiss & R. Berger (Eds.), *Posttraumatic growth and culturally competent practice: Lessons learned from around the globe* (pp. 1–14).Wiley.

Druss, R. G., & Douglas, C. J. (1988). Adaptive responses to illness and disability: Healthy denial. *General Hospital Psychiatry, 10*(3), 163–168. https://doi.org/10.1016/0163-8343(88)90015-1

Edmondson, R., & Woerner, M. H. (2019). Sociocultural foundations of wisdom. In r. J. Sternberg & J. Glück (Eds.), *Cambridge handbook of wisdom* (pp. 40–66). New York, NY: Cambridge University Press.

Ferrari, M., & Munroe, M. (2022). Coping with adversity through metaconscious wisdom. In M. Munroe & M. Ferrari (Eds.), *Post-traumatic growth to psychological well-being: Coping wisely with adversity (Lifelong learning book series, vol 30)* (pp. 67–81). Springer, Cham. https://doi.org/10.1007/978-3-031-15290-0_8

Fleeson, W. (2014). Four ways of (not) being real, and whether they are essential for post-traumatic growth. *European Journal of Personality, 28*(4), 336–337. doi:10.1002/per.1970

Frazier, P., Tennen, H., Gavian, M., Park, C., Tomich, P., & Tashiro, T. (2009). Does self-reported posttraumatic growth reflect genuine positive change?. *Psychological Science, 20*(7), 912–919. https://doi.org/10.1111/j.1467-9280.2009.02381.x

Glück, J. (2022). How MORE life experience fosters wise coping. In M. Munroe & M. Ferrari (Eds.), *Post-traumatic growth to psychological well-being: Coping wisely with adversity (Lifelong learning book series, vol 30)* (pp. 131–149). Springer Cham.

Grossmann, I. (2017). Wisdom in context. *Perspectives on Psychological Science, 12*(2), 233–257.

Hayes, J. M. (2010a). The ecology of wisdom. *Management & Marketing, 5*(1), 71–92.

Hayes, J. M. (2010b). Mapping wisdom as a complex adaptive system. *Management & Marketing, 5*(2), 19–66.

Hobfoll, S. E., Canetti-Nisim, D., Johnson, R. J., Palmieri, P. A., Varley, J. D., & Galea, S. (2008). The association of exposure, risk, and resiliency factors with PTSD among Jews and Arabs exposed to repeated acts of terrorism in Israel. *Journal of Traumatic Stress, 21*(1), 9–21. https://doi.org/10.1002/jts.20307

Janoff-Bulman, R. (1992). *Shattered assumptions.* Free Press.

Janoff-Bulman, R. (2004). Posttraumatic growth: Three explanatory models. *Psychological Inquiry, 15*(1), 30–34.

Jayawickreme, E., Infurna, F. J., Alajak, K., Blackie, L. E. R., Chopik, W. J., Chung, J., Dorfman, A., Fleeson, W., Forgeard, M. J. C., Frazier, P., Furr, R. M, Grossmann, I., Heller, A., Laceulle, O., Lucas, R. E., Luhmann, M., Luong, G., Meijer, L., McLean, K. C., . . . Zonneveld, R. (2021). Post-traumatic growth as positive personality change: Challenges, opportunities and recommendations. *Journal of Personality, 89*(1), 145–165. https://doi.org/10.31219/osf.io/uqngk

Kim, J. J., Munroe, M., Feng, Z., Morris, S., Al-Refae, M., Antonacci, R., & Ferrari, M. (2021). Personal growth and well-being in the time of COVID: An exploratory mixed-methods analysis. *Frontiers in Psychology*, *12*, 734. https://doi.org/10.3389/fpsyg.2021.648060

Koehly, L. M., Peters, J. A., Kuhn, N., Hoskins, L., Letocha, A., Kenen, R., Loud, J., & Greene, M. H. (2008). Sisters in hereditary breast and ovarian cancer families: Communal coping, social integration, and psychological well-being. *Psycho-Oncology*, *17*(8), 812–821. https://doi.org/10.1002/pon.1373.

Kong, J. D., Tekwa, E. W., & Gignoux-Wolfsohn, S. A. (2021). Social, economic, and environmental factors influencing the basic reproduction number of COVID-19 across countries. *PloS one*, *16*(6), e0252373. https://doi.org/10.1371/journal.pone.0252373

Lindstrom, C. M., Cann, A., Calhoun, L. G., & Tedeschi, R. G. (2011). The relationship of core belief challenge, rumination, disclosure, and sociocultural elements to posttraumatic growth. *Psychological Trauma: Theory, Research, Practice, and Policy*, *4*, 400–410.

Linley, P. A., & Joseph, S. (2004). Positive change following trauma and adversity: A review. *Journal of Traumatic Stress*, *17*(1), 11–21. https://doi.org/10.1023/B:JOTS.000 0014671.27856.7e

Lykes, M. B., Martín Beristain, C., & Cabrera, M. L. (2007). Political violence, impunity, and emotional climate in Maya communities. *Journal of Social Issues*, *63*(2), 369–385. https://doi.org/10.1111/j.1540-4560.2007.00514.x

Lyons, R. F., Mickelson, K. D., Sullivan, M. J., & Coyne, J. C. (1998). Coping as a communal process. *Journal of Social and Personal Relationships*, *15*(5), 579–605. https://doi.org/10.1177/0265407598155001

Magid, B., & Boothby, N. (2013). Promoting resilience in children of war. In C. Fernando & M. Ferrari (Eds.), *Handbook of resilience in children of war* (pp. 39–49). Springer.

Mannarini, T., Rizzo, M., Brodsky, A., Buckingham, S., Zhao, J., Rochira, A., & Fedi, A. (2021). The potential of psychological connectedness: Mitigating the impacts of COVID-19 through sense of community and community resilience. *Journal of Community Psychology*, 1–17. https://doi.org/10.1002/jcop.22775

Mansfield, C. D. (2022). The co-evolution of meaning-making and wisdom in processing and developmental time. In M. Munroe & M. Ferrari (Eds.), *Post-traumatic growth to psychological well-being: Coping wisely with adversity (Lifelong learning book series, vol 30)* (pp. 87–106). Springer, Cham.

McLean, K. C., & Syed, M. (2015). Personal, master, and alternative narratives: An integrative framework for understanding identity development in context. *Human Development*, *58*, 318–349. http://dx.doi.org/10.1159/000445817

McLean, K. C., Pasupathi, M., & Syed, M. (2023). Cognitive scripts and narrative identity are shaped by structures of power. *Trends in Cognitive Science*, *27*(9), 805–813.

Metatawabin, E. (2014). *Up Ghost River: A chief's journey through the turbulent waters of Native history*. Knopf (with Shimo, A.).

Muldoon, O. T., Acharya, K., Jay, S., Adhikari, K., Pettigrew, J., & Lowe, R. D. (2017). Community identity and collective efficacy: A social cure for traumatic stress in post-earthquake Nepal. *European Journal of Social Psychology*, *47*(7), 904–915. https://doi.org/10.1002/ejsp.2330

Narvaez, D. (2014). *Neurobiology and the development of human morality: Evolution, culture and wisdom*. W. W. Norton.

Neff, K. (2003). Self-compassion: An alternative conceptualization of a healthy attitude toward oneself. *Self and Identity*, *2*(2), 85–101. https://doi.org/10.1080/15298860309032

Nietzsche, F. (1889/1998). *Twilight of the idols*. Oxford University Press.

Norris, F. H., Stevens, S. P., Pfefferbaum, B., Wyche, K. F., & Pfefferbaum, R. L. (2008). Community resilience as a metaphor, theory, set of capacities, and strategy for disaster readiness. *American Journal of Community Psychology*, *41*(1-2), 127–150. https://doi.org/10.1007/s10464-007-9156-6

Páez, D., Vázquez, C., & Echeburúa, E. (2013). Trauma social, afrontamiento comunitario y crecimiento postraumático colectivo [Social trauma, community coping and collective posttraumatic growth]. In M. J. Carrasco & B. Charro Baena (Eds.), *Crisis, vulnerabilidad y superación [Crisis, vulnerability and growth]*. Universidad de Comillas.

Rhodes, A. M., & Tran, T. V. (2012). Predictors of posttraumatic stress and growth among black and white survivors of Hurricane Katrina: Does perceived quality of the governmental response matter? *Race and Social Problems*, *4*(3–4), 144–157. doi:10.1007/s12552-012-9074-6

Ricoeur, P. (1992). *Oneself as another*. University of Chicago Press.

Seow, H., McMillan, K., Civak, M., Bainbridge, D., van der Wal, A., Haanstra, C., Goldhar, J., & Winemaker, S. (2021). #Caremongering: A community-led social movement to address health and social needs during COVID-19. *PloS One*, *16*(1), e0245483. https://doi.org/10.1371/journal.pone.0245483

Spialek, M. L., & Houston, J. B. (2018). The development and initial validation of the citizen disaster communication assessment. *Communication Research*, *45*(6), 934–955. https://doi.org/10.1177/0093650217697521

Spialek, M. L., Houston, J. B., & Worley, K. C. (2019). Disaster communication, posttraumatic stress, and posttraumatic growth following Hurricane Matthew. *Journal of Health Communication*, *24*(1), 65–74. https://doi.org/10.1080/10810730.2019.1574319

Tedeschi, R. G., & Calhoun, L. G. (1995). *Trauma and transformation: Growing in the aftermath of suffering*. Sage.

Tedeschi, R. G., & Calhoun, L. G. (1996). The Posttraumatic Growth Inventory: Measuring the positive legacy of trauma. *Journal of Traumatic Stress*, *9*(3), 455–471. https://doi.org/10.1007/BF02103658

Tedeschi, R. G., & Calhoun, L. G. (2004). Posttraumatic growth: Conceptual foundations and empirical evidence. *Psychological Inquiry*, *15*(1), 1–18. https://doi.org/10.1207/s15327965pli1501_01

Tennen, H., & Affleck, G. (1998). Personality and transformation in me face of adversity. In R. G. Tedeschi, C. L. Park, & L. G. Calhoun (Eds.), *Posttraumatic growth: Positive changes in the aftermath of crisis* (pp. 65–98). Lawrence Erlbaum Associates.

Tian, X., Schrodt, P., & Carr, K. (2016). The theory of motivated information management and posttraumatic growth: Emerging adults' uncertainty management in response to an adverse life experience. *Communication Studies*, *67*(3), 280–301. https://doi.org/10.1080/10510974.2016.1164207

Tsai, C.-H. (2022). *Wisdom: A skill theory*. New York, NY: Cambridge University Press.

Tyler, M., & Rogers, J. R. (2005). A federal perspective on EAPs and emergency preparedness. *International Journal of Emergency Mental Health*, *7*(3), 179–186.

Ungar, M. (2012). Social Ecologies and Their Contribution to Resilience. In M. Ungar (Ed.), *The social ecology of resilience: A handbook of theory and practice* (pp. 13–31). Springer.

Webster, J. D. (2022). The interplay of adversity and wisdom development: The H.E.R.O.E. Model. In M. Munroe & M. Ferrari (Eds.), *Post-traumatic growth to psychological well-being: Coping wisely with adversity (Lifelong learning book series, vol 30)* (pp. 47–62). Springer Cham.

Wlodarczyk, A., Basabe, N., Páez, D., Amutio, A., García, F. E., Reyes, C., & Villagrán, L. (2016a). Positive effects of communal coping in the aftermath of a collective trauma: The case of the 2010 Chilean earthquake. *European Journal of Education and Psychology, 9*(1), 9–19. https://doi.org/10.1016/j.ejeps.2015.08.001

Wlodarczyk, A., Basabe, N., Páez, D., Reyes, C., Villagrán, L., Madariaga, C., Palacio, J., & Martínez, F. (2016b). Communal coping and posttraumatic growth in a context of natural disasters in Spain, Chile, and Colombia. *Cross-Cultural Research, 50*(4), 325–355. https://doi.org/10.1177/1069397116663857

Yanez, B. R., Stanton, A. L., Hoyt, M. A., Tennen, H., & Lechner, S. (2011). Understanding perceptions of benefit following adversity: How do distinct forms of growth relate to coping and adjustment to stressful events? *Journal of Social and Clinical Psychology, 30*, 699–721. http://dx.doi.org/10.1521/jscp.2011.30.7.699

9

Rethinking Our Lives

COVID-19 and the Narrative Imagination

Molly Andrews

Trying to write about the COVID-19 pandemic while living through it is a challenge: epistemological, psychological, and emotional. Epistemological: one of the defining characteristics about this virus is how much we do not know about it. There is not even certainty about its origins, and there is much disagreement about the best ways to try to contain it. Among the many things we do not know are how many people have it and have had it, the long-term effects of having had the virus, and what is happening behind the closed doors of many homes. Writing about and in uncertainty is hard, especially for academics who are trained to be overly assertive. Psychological: the pandemic has caused much of the world to live under quarantine, if not strict lockdown, for very protracted periods. Only several months into the pandemic, indicators already pointed to a "silent pandemic" of depression, self-harm, and suicide, especially in children and adolescents (Maker, May 2020). We do not know what the long-term consequences of the pandemic will be. We are psychologically challenged because there is no end in sight; we are thus deprived of a narrative structure to frame our experiences. Emotional: Although we might be somewhat successful at recalibrating a new daily life, still the enormity of the situation comes into full view at certain unexpected moments when we encounter details of the lives we used to live or the futures we thought we were moving toward. There are moments, and days, when we feel unanchored by the magnitude of change. Life can be overwhelming. How can this minefield of emotion be captured in scholarly writing? There are, of course, countless other dimensions which contribute to making the writing about a pandemic while living in its midst very difficult. My analysis can only be partial, an attempt to make meaning of a hurricane while trying to remain standing in its midst.

Molly Andrews, *Rethinking Our Lives* In: *Narrative in Crisis*. Edited by: Martin Dege and Irene Strasser, Oxford University Press. © Oxford University Press 2024. DOI: 10.1093/oso/9780197751756.003.0009

I first began thinking about the argument I will make in this chapter in mid-2020, when we were only a few months into the pandemic. One of the central tenets on which narrative scholarship is built is that meaning is not uncovered but made and that this is a dynamic process, forever in flux, recreated time and again and again. I have argued that we never reach a final, absolute interpretation of phenomena we seek to understand, but rather that our analyses are always provisional, offered from a particular viewpoint which will invariably change. There is "never a last word" (Andrews, 2008). This chapter is, then, temporally grounded in the political reality of Summer 2020, when Donald Trump, the Great Denier, was the President of the United States. When I first delivered this talk as a keynote address for the Psychology of Global Crisis conference, the number of persons officially recorded with the virus was 5 million (Worldometer Coronavirus Statistics) As I write, that number has multiplied by more than 50 and continues to mount. How, then, can one write about something which is very much still in motion and whose fallout is likely to dominate our lives for many years to come?

Millions of people have already died, and more will continue to do so; the challenge before us as academics is to see if there is anything at all that we can contribute to help make sense of the new world in which we now find ourselves. What I offer here, then, are thoughts from the field; where this pandemic journey is taking us still remains to be seen.

Although it is sometimes said these days that what we are experiencing is "unimaginable," I believe that our imagination is the very muscle which might be able to give us insight into the present pandemonium. In the opening pages of my book *Narrative Imagination and Everyday Life,* I argued that "The coupling of narrative and imagination brings into focus: (1) the salience of, and dynamic nature of, the temporal; (2) a mediation between the real and the not-real and the not-yet-real; and (3) the complexity of the construction of 'the other.'" In this chapter, I use this framework to analyse the challenge of narrating the COVID-19 pandemic.

Fluid Temporality: "Time Traveling" During the Pandemic

Narrative scholars have long argued for a dynamic construction of time, adherents of Heraclitus's view that "No man ever steps in the same river twice, for it's not the same river, and he's not the same man." Time does not stand still. Rather, the past, present, and future are constantly woven and rewoven into one another, recasting and being recast anew in light of the ever-changing present. Things which happened in the past suddenly become imbued with a new significance, shedding light not only on the present but on the very way in which we view the past. Our sense of what lies ahead is also in constant flux as the unfolding present creates new possibilities while it erases others. The paths that lie before us hold both dreams and nightmares of a world which might be ours.

Elsewhere I have described this temporal fluidity as "time traveling":

> We are forever revisiting our pasts, in light of changing circumstances of the present, and in so doing, our vision for the future is reconstituted. Not only can we time travel, but we do it all the time. We must. We constantly move backwards and forwards in our mind's eye, and it is this movement which is a key stimulus behind our development. We learn from our pasts, not only as things happen, but as we reflect back on experience, in light of subsequent unfoldings. We routinely revisit moments in our lives where we now realise that, had we chosen a different path, things would have turned out very differently. (Andrews, 2014, p. 3)

It is hard to think of a context which illustrates this time-traveling more dramatically than that of a pandemic.

By April 2020, within weeks of the World Health Organization declaring COVID-19 a pandemic, about half of the world's population was under some form of lockdown; eventually, this became a "global lockdown" (though a few countries did not adopt this policy.) While historically there have been many pandemics (already five in this relatively new century alone), never has such a great proportion of the world's population simultaneously been in lockdown (Onyeaka et al., 2021). Thus, this was a shared phenomenon, but one which was experienced alone or with a very limited group of people. Lockdown poses innumerable challenges; the one which concerns us here is the profoundly altered sense of time which it occasioned. The days no longer were framed by their usual structure, which habitually marks one's sense of the passage of time itself. Yesterday, last week, last month blurred into one another. Days seemed to pass both quickly and slowly. More accurately, they were marked by achronicity, and we tried to navigate our lives as best we could in this new-found sense of living outside of time. We relied on our memories to bring us back to a known, identifiable past; things one did and didn't do, enjoyments taken and forestalled, gatherings with others, trips, celebrations, bike rides, concerts. Had we known then what we later came to know about the future that was awaiting us, might we have made different choices?

The past, newly reconstructed, became littered with crossroads pregnant with questions of "what if"? This was true not only for individuals but, critically, also for societies. What if we had taken the risk of the virus more seriously earlier? In the United Kingdom, for instance, Neil Ferguson, the head of the outbreak modeling group at Imperial College London, stated that the unusually high death toll in the country would have been halved had lockdown regulations been introduced only one week earlier (ABC News, June 10, 2020). (The United Kingdom implemented these measures later than most European countries, on March 23). Finland, in contrast, looked to its neighbor Sweden that did not impose a quarantine on its population and counted the Finnish deaths that had been avoided by choosing an early shutdown of the country. Three months into the pandemic, a senior researcher at the Finnish Institute for Health and Welfare (THL) reported that "had Finland followed Sweden's example in the battle against the new coronavirus, its death toll from the virus would already stand at 2,524 [as opposed to 301 at time of statement.] translating to the loss of 22,269 life-years" (*Helsinki Times,* June 11, 2020).

The case of the United States, with its exceptionally high loss of human life, is particularly marked. In contrast to Trump's claims that Obama had left "no game plan" for a pandemic, in fact, Obama's National Security Council left the incoming president a 69-page document—40 pages plus appendices—called "Playbook for Early Response to High-Consequence Emerging Infectious Disease Threats and Biological Incidents." The playbook "explicitly lists novel coronaviruses as one of the kinds of pathogens that could require a major response" and "addresses issues like testing, funding, personal protective equipment, emergency declarations, border control measures, diplomacy, the use of the military, public communication, even mortuary services" (Dale, May 2020). It is not clear if anyone in the Trump administration ever read the playbook. In addition to the playbook, "outgoing senior Obama officials also led an in-person pandemic response exercise for senior incoming Trump officials in January 2017" (Dale, May 2020). There is no evidence to suggest that any of this early preparedness was taken seriously by the Trump administration. On the contrary. By May 2018, only four months into office, Trump closed down the National Security Council's pandemic response team, which had been charged with preparing for "when, not if, another pandemic would hit the nation." (ABC News, March 14, 2020). It seems fair to say that Trump's White House demonstrated willful blindness to the risks which lay in store.

There are other examples of this (*New York Times*, March 19, 2020). Between January and August 2019, a simulation exercise called "Crimson Contagion" was run by the Department of Health and Human Services. The report which was delivered to the White House in October described the federal government as "underfunded, underprepared and uncoordinated . . . for a life-or-death battle with a virus for which no treatment existed." The following month, at the end of November 2019, the National Center for Medical Intelligence informed the White House that they had detected unusual activity in China's Wuhan region. The report was based on wire and computer intercepts combined with satellite images. "Analysts concluded it could be a cataclysmic event." The White House appeared to take no notice. Finally, between early January and February, when the existence of the virus in China was already publicly known, the White House received a dozen intelligence briefings "warning of the threat of a pandemic." On February 27, the Senate Intelligence Committee concluded that the virus, far from being like the common flu, was "probably more akin to the 1918 pandemic." It is very difficult not to look back on the determined way in which these series of clear warnings were systematically ignored and not to be consumed with grief over the needless loss of life that resulted from inaction, a sense that there had been other alternatives available to us in the past.

Another example of the past being revisited and reconstructed in light of prevailing circumstances can be seen in the current fascination with past pandemics. Once the thing of a long ago and far away history, the pandemic has brought horrors of yesteryear much closer to home. As hot spots of the pandemic struggled to bury their dead, there was a certain resonance with days of old in which mass graves were dug in the heart of London to accommodate the dramatic increase in bodies. According to Catharine Arnold (2007), author of *Necropolis: London and Its Dead*, the Black Death of 1348 killed between a third and a half of London's population in an 18-month period. (Only now have I become aware of the origins of the name Pitfield Street—where trenches were dug to throw the corpses during the Black Plague—which lies at the corner of my own street in London.) Especially people in the Global North had come to regard those times as long gone, and indeed they had very little historical consciousness of their existence, regarding them rather as simply the stuff of which nightmares are made. The arrival of COVID-19 changed that. By mid-May 2020, for instance, John Barry's *The Great Influenza: The Story of the Deadliest Pandemic in History*, published in 2005, had already been on the *New York Times* bestseller list for eight weeks.

The pandemic has caused us not only to revisit the past but to apply a new lens to our present lives. The phrase "the new normal" is batted around as people acknowledge that what had once seemed extraordinary rather quickly became the everyday and, conversely, that many habitual practices which we used to take for granted appear to be suspended indefinitely. This rupture of the everyday has caused many to experience the pandemic as a time of crisis, not only for the world at large but for themselves personally. The radical cessation of the world as we knew it caused us to question things we had once taken for granted. Especially for young people, but also for others, there is an overwhelming sense that this present life is not the world we thought we were moving toward. We are called upon to reimagine our lives from the most intimate to the most public spaces.

The third component of the time-traveling journey occasioned by the pandemic is oriented toward the future. If we are not living the future life we thought we had been moving towards in the past, it is most certainly true that it is now demanded of us that we rethink our futures. The uncertainty produced by the pandemic and the rupture of our everyday lives have altered not only the assumptions which guide our movements in the world but created in our mind's eye new fears and possibilities for our futures. In the decade prior to the onslaught of COVID-19, there developed a growing literature on the sociology of the future seeking not to illuminate "what is, but to create what is to become" (Gergen, 2015, p. 294). Sools's (2020) innovative methodology of writing letters to oneself from an imagined future self reflects a similar focus. But even these scholars, with their forward-looking lenses, did not and could not anchor their research in a present world of a global pandemic; these very conscious attempts at future imaginings belong to a pre-pandemic moment. Rebecca Solnit comments that we must find "another version of who we are . . . equipping ourselves for an unanticipated world" (Solnit, 2020).

Thus it is that we time-travel, back and forth and back again, interweaving different temporalities, thinking of a world that at one time might have been, but whose possibility is no longer, the crises averted or accentuated by actions taken irretrievably, the new possible futures which might save or destroy us.

All the while, our narrative imaginations are working overtime, storying different scenarios in light of our dramatically altered circumstances of living in these pandemic times. The pandemic is not "unimaginable" but rather demands a fundamental reimagining of who we are, who we have been, and who we might become.

Mediating Between the Real, the Not-Real, and the Not-Yet Real

One of the challenges of the current situation is that of differentiating between what is real—in terms of both what is known and what is knowable—what is false, and what is not currently real but could become so. We are not used to dealing with this level of uncertainty in virtually all aspects of our lives. Moreover, recent years have witnessed an increasing cynicism toward "expert opinion." Just under three weeks before the United Kingdom had its referendum vote on Brexit, Michael Gove, then Justice Secretary, when asked to name any economists who backed the plan for Britain to exit from the European Union, responded, "people in this country have had enough of experts" (*Financial Times,* June 2016). There are traces of this post-expert leaning during this COVID-19 pandemic. An example of this was the fact that Donald Trump appointed Vice President Mike Pence to head his coronavirus response team, while the president's son-in-law, Jared Kushner, created his own shadow task force. Neither man had scientific background and appeared to have been selected largely because of their ideological approaches. Trump, initially casting himself as a wartime president, abandoned his daily press meetings when his suggestions—such as injecting disinfectant as a precaution against the virus—had a negative impact on his popularity ratings. Anthony Fauci, the Director of the National Institute of Allergy and Infectious Disease, who at the beginning of the pandemic was the public voice of scientific reason, became less visible as the months wore on. Despite Trump's best efforts at minimalizing the losses suffered and what that portended for the future, Fauci confessed on June 9, 2020, "Now we have something that turned out to be my worst nightmare. In the period of four months, it has devastated the world. It just took over the planet. And it isn't over yet" (CNBC, June 2020). In early 2022, the end is still not in sight.

At the time of writing, there have been more than 5 million deaths (Worldometer Coronavirus Statistics). The virus has brought in its wake other new realities: in some places, there has been a rise in trade unionism (as workers protested at places like Amazon for being required to carry on as key workers—delivering vital goods such as vibrators—rather than sheltering at home; see *The Guardian,* 2020); the early release of short-term prisoners (by the first week of May 2020, Scotland sanctioned the release of up to 450 prisoners upon the virus-related death of a prison officer); sheltering of the homeless in hotels (such as Los Angeles' Project Roomkey, with London, Paris, Berlin, and Tokyo among other cities following their example and developing similar pilot programs (Solnit, 2020); and the granting of temporary citizenship and/or work permits to migrants and asylum seekers in Portugal and Italy.

Other realities of the pandemic have included a severe rollback on citizens' rights in some countries. With the increase in digital surveillance, the restriction on public gathering; the high degree of governmental control over the movement of people; the dissemination (and sometimes manipulation) of information; the silencing and even imprisoning of critics, including some journalists; the imposition of indefinite states of emergency; and other indicators of the suspension of democratic norms have meant that activists such as Evan Mawarire from Zimbabwe describe the virus as "a gift to totalitarian governments" (Covidcon, 2020). (For more information on these alarming developments, visit the COVID-19 Civic Freedom Tracker, https://www.icnl.org/covid19tracker/; see International Centre for Not-for-Profit Law, 2020.) As Kenneth Roth, Executive Director of Human Rights Watch, summarized

> There is no question these are extraordinary times. International human rights law permits restrictions on liberty in times of national emergency that are necessary and proportionate. But we should be very wary of leaders who exploit this crisis to serve their political ends. They are jeopardizing both democracy and our health. (Roth, 2020)

Clearly, the realities of the pandemic are complex and far-reaching. As commented in the opening of this chapter, they are also difficult to capture because the pace of change is exceptionally swift. Indeed, it is difficult to think of any aspect of life which is untouched by the exceptional conditions created and/or accentuated by the pandemic.

One of the greatest impediments to fighting the spread of the virus has been the proliferation of the "not-real" information about it, which has been systematically disseminated by some governments. Here, I focus on the example of Donald Trump, who was President of the United States in the critical first few months of the pandemic. While his case is a dramatic one in terms of the willful blindness which characterized his leadership, he is by no means alone on the stage of world leaders who refused to acknowledge the reality of the pandemic and failed to take the necessary precautions to protect their people. Here, Trump stands in the company of Bolsonaro, Modi, Putin, and others. But, for the purposes of this chapter, I focus on Trump as the leader of the most powerful country in the world, which has nonetheless suffered the greatest loss of life from the pandemic. Despite this reality, Donald Trump characterized the virus as "a hoax" and "a conspiracy," describing it as "contained," "unique in history," "no worse than the seasonal flu," and other falsehoods. All of this misinformation played a vital role in efforts to combat the exponential growth of COVID-19 in the early months of the virus when the possibility for its containment was greatest. Trump's denial of any shortage of personal protective equipment (PPE) and of tests contributed to what Barack Obama described as "the absolute chaotic disaster" of Trump's response to the coronavirus (CNN News, May 2020).

Many Trump supporters followed the President's lead, doubting the severity of the virus and demanding an early lifting of the restrictions imposed by the quarantine. As one supporter tweeted beneath a photo of a young man with muscular, tanned arms folded across his chest: "All the people who are placing themselves under 'self-quarantine' are posers looking for a few cheap headlines. Stop being a baby and go to the gym. Obesity is the real pandemic" (Coppins, March 2020).

In the spring of 2020, when the President should have been focusing all of his efforts on fighting the spread of the virus, he repeatedly cast doubt on the seriousness of the situation, offering instead a baseless assurance which he hoped would help to secure his re-election the following November. For months, he ambushed the people of the United States with disinformation which he hoped would cause the gathering clouds to disperse.

- "We have it totally under control. It's one person coming in from China, and we have it under control. It's going to be just fine." (CNBC, January 22, 2020)
- "We're going to be pretty soon at only five people. And we could be at just one or two people over the next short period of time. So we've had very good luck." (White House Press Briefings, February 26, 2020)

- "It's going to disappear. One day—it's like a miracle—it will disappear." (CNN, February 27, 2020)
- "I just think this is something . . . that you can never really think is going to happen. . . . It's an unforeseen problem. . . . What a problem. Came out of nowhere." (MSNBC, March 6, 2020)
- Coronavirus "blind-sided the world" (CNN, March 9, 2020)
- "I would view it as something that just surprised the whole world. . . . So there's never been anything like this in history. There's never been. . . . And nobody's ever seen anything like this." (*The Washington Post*, March 19, 2020)

Assurance after assurance after assurance. Meanwhile, the death toll continued to spike.

In complete contrast to Trump's repeated misrepresentations, this is not the first pandemic the world has ever experienced, nor did it come as a surprise to anyone who knew about epidemiology or took the time to read reports prepared by scientists about the level of risk they posed. One cannot overestimate the negative impact such blatant falsehoods wielded over public understanding and, ultimately, the spread of the virus.

Harvard psychiatrist John Mack (1984) described "resistances to knowing" exhibited by people who turned their heads away from learning about the nuclear threat and its potential widespread fatal consequences. In a similar vein, Trump exhibited a steadfast determination not to know about the existence of the virus. Time after time after time, there were moments when the president was presented with critical information about the potential for, and later the existence of, the outbreak of the virus. As demonstrated earlier in this chapter, again and again, he turned away, embracing a willful ignorance.

The third and final strand of Trump's embracing of the "not-real" with regards to the pandemic was his overt and unmerited optimism about the spread of the virus despite the extraordinary death toll in the United States. Trump appeared to adopt the attitude that if he acted as if things were going well, they would be perceived as being so. Thus he made the following claims, evaluating his own performance and how he allegedly believed the rest of the world regarded the way in which the United States dealt with the virus in those critical first few months:

- "A great success story." (CNN, April 29, 2020)
- "We did a spectacular job," rating his handling of the disease "I'd rate it a 10." (CNN, April 30, 2020)

- "We've done a great job." (CNN, May 1, 2020)
- "We're opening up our country again. And this is what we're doing. And I'll tell you, the whole world is excited watching us because we're leading the world." (White House Press Briefings, May 5, 2020)
- "For those people that have lost somebody . . . nothing can ever happen that's gonna replace that. . . . . From an economic standpoint, purely an economic standpoint, I think next year's potentially gonna be one of the best years we've ever had." (White House Press Briefings, May 6, 2020)
- "All throughout the country, the numbers are coming down rapidly." (White House Press Briefings, May 11, 2020)

It is not surprising that the effect of this magical thinking was simply to fan the explosion of the contagion.

In Jean-Paul Sartre's *The Psychology of Imagination*, he identifies two different sorts of futures: "the one is but the temporal ground on which my present perception develops, the other is posited for itself as *that which is not yet*" (1940/1972, p. 211). The "not-yet-real" holds particular relevance in these pandemic times as different possible futures line themselves up in our long-term vision depending on what decisions of action or inaction are made in the current moment. This framing has been instrumental in terms of trying to predict how the virus will behave and what measures are most effective in combatting it. Generally, those countries where the virus occurred earliest tended to face the most significant challenge to controlling its spread. In Europe, for instance, Italy and Spain were initially the hardest hit. Some countries (e.g., France, Germany, most of Scandinavia) heeded the warning that imposing an early quarantine would increase the chances of a successful strategy. The general sense was that if drastic measures were not adopted urgently, then they could make themselves vulnerable to becoming "like Italy or Spain," And indeed those countries which took those measures in a timely fashion tended to fare better—at least in the first waves of the virus—than countries such as the United Kingdom and Sweden, which, for different reasons, did not do so.

Narrative Imagination and Imagining "the Other"

The third and final point regarding the vital relationship between narrative and imagination brings into focus the challenge of imagining life from a different point of view. Just as the pandemic has forced us to question who we are when those performative aspects of our life that formed the basis of our "everyday" have been stripped away, so, too, we are now cast into a position of questioning our position vis á vis those who we constitute as "other." I have written earlier about this dynamic perspective-taking.

> How and what one perceives and understands about one's own life is always connected to one's view of others. Who am I (and who are "us") invariably invites the question of who are "they" (or other). This construction of self and other is ongoing, and draws equally on (situated) knowledge and imagination, reaching out not only to the future (aspirations and fears), but deeply rooted in our pasts (sometimes acknowledged, sometimes hidden). How one comes to think of oneself in relation to others and to negotiate the space between them is not only the basis of much moral philosophy, but is something with which we are confronted every day of our lives. The challenge is practical and ethical in equal parts, and at its heart is the question of who and how we are in the world. (Andrews, 2014, pp. 8–9)

The pandemic has caused some people to become newly conscious of their own vulnerability; a world which had once seemed stable has become transformed into a sea of risk and precarity, be it in terms of health, employment, social engagement, or a number of other dimensions. Historically, those with privilege in the Global North have tended to regard massive outbreaks of disease as being someone else's story, not theirs. Even in recent decades, the alphabet of epidemics (SARS, MERS, ZIKA, Ebola, AIDS) has failed to penetrate the psychological armor protecting the illusion of immunity. But now, this story of invincibility has been replaced by one of susceptibility. In the early weeks of the outbreak in the United Kingdom, much was made of the fact that the heir to the throne, Prince Charles, and Prime Minister Boris Johnson had both fallen victim to the virus. A mantra developed: "We are all in this together." But that chorus quieted as it soon became abundantly clear that certain populations were more prone to getting COVID-19 than others. As *Guardian* journalist Owen Jones wrote,

> save us the platitudes of coronavirus as the great leveller; abandon this sickly myth that we are all in this together. For some, this is a time of grand inconvenience, of undoubted stress, of a self-evident loss of freedom. For others, this is both a national and personal disaster, a present defined by turmoil and of futures snatched away. (Jones, April 2020)

Far from being a "great leveler," the pandemic has been "an amplifier of existing inequalities, injustices and insecurities" (Jones, April 2020).

For some people of privilege, a vulnerability that pre-pandemic seemed "unimaginable" became transformed into something all too real. For others, however, living under conditions of fundamental insecurity and uncertainty was all too easily imaginable; there are many for whom the pandemic has not been the most challenging experience they have had to endure. Aditya Chakrobortty writes of his recently deceased mother's early life.

> They were plunged close to poverty, then saw their family land in East Bengal disappear after partition. Even now, as our world is turned upside down, it is worth remembering that some among us have lived through far worse. (Chakrobortty, 2020)

While the pandemic has produced and been produced by global crises, it has revealed and exacerbated deep chasms of inequality, which will only grow. Crisis heaped upon crisis, heaped upon crisis. The tentacles of change stretch far beyond our restricted field of vision. One of our greatest challenges is "to understand this moment, what it might require of us, and what it might make possible" (Solnit, 2020).

Living in this pandemic moment, with all the suffering in its wake, there is a distant hope that we will not only come through this hard journey, but that we will learn something from it. The interconnectedness of our world, across space and time, has been demonstrated to us in Technicolor. We sit at a "hinge in history" (Summers, 2020) with the outcome still to be determined. We cannot go back to that lethal cocktail of circumstances and practices which led us, inevitably it now seems, to this dark hour, yet we struggle to move forward. "Historically, pandemics have forced humans to break with the past and imagine their world anew," Arundhati Roy (April 2020) writes.

> This one is no different. It is a portal, a gateway between one world and the next. We can choose to walk through it, dragging the carcasses of our prejudice and hatred, our avarice, our data banks and dead ideas, our dead rivers and smoky skies behind us. Or we can walk through lightly, with little luggage, ready to imagine another world. And ready to fight for it. (Roy, 2020)

Whether or not we will be equal to this task is yet to be seen.

References

ABC News. (March 14, 2020). Trump disbanded NSC pandemic unit that experts had praised https://abcnews.go.com/Politics/wireStory/trump-disbanded-nsc-pandemic-unit-experts-praised-69594177

ABC News. (June 10, 2020). UK coronavirus deaths could have been cut by half if lockdown came earlier, top epidemiologist says. https://www.abc.net.au/news/2020-06-11/uk-deaths-could-have-been-cut-by- half-if-lockdown-came-earlier/12342560

Andrews, M. (2008). Never the last word: Narrative research and secondary analysis. In C. Squire, M. Tamboukou, & M. Andrews (Eds.), *Doing narrative research*. Sage.

Andrews, M. (2014). *Narrative imagination and everyday life*. Oxford University Press.

Arnold, C. (2007). *Necropolis: London and its dead*. Simon and Schuster.

Barry, J. (2005). *The great influenza: the story of the deadliest pandemic in history*. Penguin Books.

Chakrobortty, A. (April 30, 2020). What my mother's glorious life taught me about Britain today. *The Guardian*. https://www.theguardian.com/commentisfree/2020/apr/30/my-mother-life- british-society-coronavirus

CNBC. (January 22, 2020). Trump struggles to explain why he disbanded his global health team https://www.msnbc.com/rachel-maddow-show/trump-struggles- explain-why-he-disbanded-his-global-health-team-n1153221

CNBC. (June 9, 2020). Dr. Anthony Fauci says coronavirus turned "out to be my worst nightmare" and it "isn't over." https://www.cnbc.com/2020/06/09/dr-anthony- fauci-says-coronavirus-turned-out-to-be-my-worst-nightmare-and-it-isnt- over.html

CNN. (February 27, 2020). Trump says coronavirus will "disappear" eventually. https://edition.cnn.com/2020/02/27/politics/trump-coronavirus- disappear/index.html

CNN. (March 9, 2020). March 9 coronavirus news. https://edition.cnn.com/asia/live-news/coronavirus-outbreak-03-09-20-intl- hnk/h_74b40cb6d19ef01601b094a1c8c94 aaa

CNN. (April 29, 2020). Kushner calls US coronavirus response a "success story" as cases hit 1 million. https://edition.cnn.com/2020/04/29/politics/jared-kushner-coronavirus-success-story/index.html

CNN. (May 1, 2020). Trump on handling of coronavirus: "I think we've done a great job." https://edition.cnn.com/2020/05/01/world/meanwhile-in-america-may- 1/index.html

CNN. (May 9, 2020). Obama says White House response to coronavirus has been "absolute chaotic disaster." https://edition.cnn.com/2020/05/09/politics/obama-trump-coronavirus- response-flynn-case/index.html

Coppins, M. (March 12, 2020). Twitter. https://twitter.com/mckaycoppins/status/1237 915100234813440/photo/1

Covidcon Virtual Conference. (2020, April 13–14). https://covidcon.org/

Dale, D., CNN.Com Wire Service (May 12, 2020). Fact check: Obama left Trump a pandemic response playbook. https://www.mercurynews.com/2020/05/12/fact-check-obama-left-trump-a- pandemic-response-playbook/

Financial Times. (June 3, 2016). Britain has had enough of experts, says Gove. https://www.ft.com/content/3be49734-29cb-11e6-83e4-abc22d5d108c

Gergen, K. (2015). From mirroring to world-making: Research as future forming *Journal for the Theory of Social Behaviour*, 45(3), 287–310.

The Guardian. (April 21, 2020). Hundreds of Amazon warehouse workers to call in sick in Coronavirus protest. https://www.theguardian.com/technology/2020/apr/20/amazon-warehouse-workers-sickout-coronavirus

Helsinki Times. (June 11, 2020). THL: Over 2,500 would've already died had Finland gone down same road as Sweden. https://www.helsinkitimes.fi/finland/finland- news/domestic/17764-thl-over-2-500-would-ve-already-died-had-finland- gone-down-same-road-as-sweden.html

International Centre for Not-for-Profit Law and European Centre for Not-for-Profit Law. (2020). COVID-19 civic freedom tracker. https://www.icnl.org/covid19tracker/?location=&issue=10&date=&type=

Jones, O. (April 9, 2020). Coronavirus is not some great leveler: It is exacerbating inequality right now. *The Guardian.* https://www.theguardian.com/commentisfree/2020/apr/09/coronavirus- inequality-managers-zoom-cleaners-offices

Mack, J. (1984). Resistances to knowing in the nuclear age. *Harvard Educational Review, 54*(3), 260–271.

Maker, A. (May 21, 2020). The silent pandemic: Depression, self-harm and suicide. *Psychology Today.* https://www.psychologytoday.com/us/blog/helping- kids-cope/202005/the-silent-pandemic-depression-self-harm-and-suicide

MSNBC. (March 6, 2020). Trump struggles to explain why he disbanded his global health team. https://www.msnbc.com/rachel-maddow-show/trump-struggles-explain- why-he-disbanded-his-global-health-team-n1153221

New York Times. (March 19, 2020). Before virus outbreak, as cascade of warning went unheeded. https://www.nytimes.com/2020/03/19/us/politics/trump- coronavirus-outbreak.html

Onyeakam, H., Anumudu, C. K., Al-Sharify, S. T., Egele-Godswill, E., & Mbaegbu, P. (2021). Covid-19 pandemic: A review of the global lockdown and its far-reaching effects. *Science Progress, 24*(2). https://doi.org/10.1177/00368504211019854.

Roth, K. (April 3, 2020). How authoritarians are exploiting the COVID-19 crisis to grab power. https://www.hrw.org/news/2020/04/03/how-authoritarians-are- exploiting-covid-19-crisis-grab-power

Roy, A. (April 3, 2020). The pandemic is a portal. *Financial Times.* https://www.ft.com/content/10d8f5e8-74eb-11ea-95fe-fcd274e920ca

Sartre, J. P. (1940/1972). *The psychology of imagination.* Methuen.

Solnit, R. (April 7, 2020). The impossible has already happened: What coronavirus can teach us about hope. *The Guardian.* https://www.theguardian.com/world/2020/apr/07/what-coronavirus-can- teach-us-about-hope-rebecca-solnit

Sools, A. (2020). Back from the future: A narrative approach to study the imagination of personal futures. *International Journal of Social Research Methodology, 23*(4), 451–465.

Summers, L. (May 14, 2020). COVID-19 looks like a hinge in history. *Financial Times.* https://www.ft.com/content/de643ae8-9527-11ea-899a-f62a20d54625

Washington Post. (March 19, 2020). Trump keeps saying "nobody" could have foreseen coronavirus. We keep finding out about new warning signs. https://www.washingtonpost.com/politics/2020/03/19/trump-keeps-saying- nobody-could-have-foreseen-coronavirus-we-keep-finding-out-about-new- warning-signs/

Washington Post. (April 27, 2020). The President´s intelligence briefing book repeatedly cited virus threat. https://www.washingtonpost.com/national- security/

presidents-intelligence-briefing-book-repeatedly-cited-virus-   threat/2020/04/27/ca66949a-8885-11ea-ac8a-fe9b8088e101_story.html

White House Press Briefings. (February 26, 2020). Remarks by President Trump, Vice President Pence, and members of the coronavirus task force in press conference. https://www.whitehouse.gov/briefings-statements/remarks-   president-trump-vice-president-pence-members-coronavirus-task-force-press- conference/

White House Press Briefings. (May 5, 2020). Remarks by President Trump before Marine One departure. https://www.whitehouse.gov/briefings-statements/rema rks- president-trump-marine-one-departure-89/

White House Press Briefings. (May 6, 2020). Remarks by President Trump in roundtable discussion on supporting Native Americans in Phoenix, AZ. https://www.whitehouse.gov/briefings-statements/remarks-president-trump-roundtable-discussion-supporting-native-americans-phoenix-az/

White House Press Briefings. (May 11, 2020). Remarks by President Trump in a press briefing on COVID-19 testing. https://www.whitehouse.gov/briefings- statements/remarks-president-trump-press-briefing-covid-19-testing/

Worldometer—Coronavirus Statistics https://www.worldometers.info/coronavirus/

10

The Self and Its Crises

Jens Brockmeier

One

Much has been written on COVID-19. Not only has the pandemic become a worldwide health catastrophe, but it is also a common topic in many usually unconnected areas, from medicine and the sciences to politics, philosophy, history, literature, art, and journalism—and the list goes on. Many different vocabularies have been applied, many names used to capture the appearance of the coronavirus and its variants. But there is not only the virus pervading all these discourses; another concept is the self. This is puzzling enough because the self is originally a philosophical and psychological construct—what that is I will explain in a moment—that stems from a theoretical milieu not commonly at the center of worldwide attention.

However, this is not really surprising. The concept of the self—especially, of the self viewed as a substantial, self-contained, and self-reflexive entity—is a time-honored battle horse. Often employed interchangeably with identity, subjectivity, and ego, it has managed to survive centuries of combat and crisis. Why should it not be used to understand a contemporary virus or, more precisely, its target? Take psychology. Given the individualistic perspective of much of psychological research and intervention, it is "best practice" to localize the self in the middle of things. After all, the self is the fundamental category, "the immediate datum in psychology," as postulated by one of the discipline's founding fathers, William James (1880/1950, p. 226).

More perplexing is a particular understanding of the self and its appearances in view of the pandemic that is insinuated by terms like "the modern self," "the Western self," the "threatened self," "the attacked self," or simply "our self." In this understanding, the self is taken for granted as a given being, a manifest entity on the same ontological level as, well, the coronavirus. Even the plain semantics underlying this ontological equalization are widespread: there is a self (which in this context is almost congruent to what

Jens Brockmeier, *The Self and Its Crises* In: *Narrative in Crisis*. Edited by: Martin Dege and Irene Strasser, Oxford University Press. © Oxford University Press 2024. DOI: 10.1093/oso/9780197751756.003.0010 we usually call a "person"), and there is a crisis; and then the self is affected by the crisis and, perhaps, by the way the crisis is managed—and it reacts through a crisis. Perhaps because this formula is so simple and so often repeated it appears logical or at least plausible.

Of course, there are a variety of more dramatic versions of the self in crisis. Some reflect pathological and clinical aspects of the pandemic. For example, many studies on the crises of the self during or after COVID-19 deal with depression, anxiety, helplessness, alcohol and drug abuse, posttraumatic stress disorder, and strokes—in various countries and populations. There are works on psychoses in individuals living under conditions of lockdown and quarantine. One-third of those affected by COVID-19 will suffer from neurological and psychiatric long-term symptoms. Other versions of the self in crisis are more political and sociological, emphasizing experiences of uncertainty, powerlessness, loss of independence, control, freedom, sovereignty.

Despite the differentiation and complexity that all these experiences add to the picture, what underlies many of them are highly problematic assumptions. First of all, that there is *a* self, an independent, stable, and functioning entity that, second, has come under heavy attack—like a vital organism comes under attack when a coronavirus is inhaled and infects lung tissue, comparable to an intruding "micro-biotic terrorist," as an epidemiologist called the virus. But before this, before the attack, the organism—like the self—was functional. It worked more or less well, perhaps even in a healthy fashion. And it will again do so once the attack is warded off, the intruder is destroyed, and the organism—like the self—is re-established in its integrity.

Two

There is a long tradition of philosophical and psychological thinking that has repudiated exactly this idea of the self as an autonomous entity, a bastion of the ego that defends its sovereignty against hostile intruders. Many studies have critically reviewed the history of this idea, rejecting it as a valid model of human self and identity. Nevertheless, it seems that this idea is not only a veteran battle horse; it also is a comeback kid. It returns again and again, irrespective of all defeats it has already suffered. As a cultural figure, the idea of a substantial self reappears especially in times of crisis, catastrophe, and disaster—in scenarios, that is, that can be depicted in tropes which comprise an external attacker. The self in crisis is the self attacked. As if the attack on the self in the first place confirms the idea of the self. If an entity can be attacked, it ostensibly must exist.

It has often been observed that psychological concepts are particularly prone to being substantialized. Kurt Danziger (1990) identified a tendency permeating psychology, from its beginning, to ontologize its basic assumptions about human existence by reifying them. James's writings offered only one, although momentous, example of how the self could turn into that self-contained "immediate datum" of psychology. Apart from the period of dominance of behaviorism in America, there has been an influential psychology of the self ever since.

Psychology might be particularly susceptible to this conceptual problem. For Klaus Holzkamp (2013), personality is a paradigmatic example of this—as is the self, Rom Harré (1998) pointed out. The problem, however, is more general. Many concepts coagulate and solidify the phenomena they seek to articulate. In principle, concepts are meant to bring order and structure to chaos; but what if it is the very nature of the phenomena at stake that they are in constant transformation? There is a danger that concepts domesticate rather than help envision the chaos and the mess, the vagueness, ambiguity, and contingency that are part of human life, not to mention human imagination. Therefore, artists have always tried to avoid this imposition; in fact, they are afraid of the moment in which "the chaos is used up," Berthold Brecht remarked, because, as he added, "it is the best of time" (1971, p. 163).

Given conducive conditions, the concepts of the self are like avatars that mutate into human characters. To understand this mutation, cultural narratology might help. Take premodern myths, which are comparable tropical figures. Originally oral narrative forms and practices, many mythical figures transformed and took on a robust, lifelike gestalt, reappearing for centuries and millennia in literature, philosophy, religion, art, and everyday imagination. Much of this mythical substantializing happens in storied forms. In the life of a culture, there is abundant narrative material. The vaguer it is, the more it serves as rough material for such transformation. Take this one: the self leads a peaceful and idyllic life, but then a challenger emerges, out of the blue, or more precisely, out of an anonymous shop in a remote Chinese marketplace, a somehow archaic wet market. There might be bats involved, dogs, and rats and—who knows—early evolutionary creatures. Perhaps also undercover agents, scientists engaged in secret operations. From the beginning, this challenger, the enemy, has a name, "coronavirus." I wonder if a marketing agency would have been able to come up with something more compelling.

Now we have the two protagonists needed for many stories told by psychologists, but also by epidemiologists, political commentators, and countless other pundits: Corona and the self in crisis. At this point it is not at all surprising to read in one of these stories, written by a psychologist, the question: "How can such a tiny virus become so powerful, giving such a massive narcissistic blow to the modern self?"

Three

It is helpful to remember that the term "narcissistic blow" has a venerable history in psychology. In 1917, Sigmund Freud distinguished three narcissistic injuries (or wounds or scars) to characterize events that challenge the narcissism, or more generically, the self-worth of a person or group of people (Freud, 1955). Freud argued that the "general narcissism" of the Western self experienced three fundamental injuries. These humiliations of humans' self-worth came in the wake of three scientific discoveries: that of Copernicus, according to which we are not in the center of the universe after all; that of Darwin who showed that we are not of godly origin but evolved in the same way as apes and, in fact, viruses. And finally, Freud referred to the psychoanalytical discovery of the unconscious, the fact that we are not masters in our own house.

While Freud has often been criticized for individualizing and biologizing certain aspects of human psychology, his view of the historical dimension of the Western self and the various crises it experienced can be understood as an attempt to culturally localize these crises beyond the individual domain. I imagine that he would have localized the COVID pandemic and its impact on the "general narcissism" of the Western self on the same cultural map. Freud might have neglected many other sociohistorical aspects, but it is remarkable that, at a time—we are in the early 20th century—when universalist claims of Western psychology and philosophy were generally taken for granted, he conceived of the idea of the self as taking shape, from the beginning, as a culturally specific psychological construct, a construct of crisis.

And Freud was not the only one. There has been a long-standing tradition in Western thinking addressing issues of human existence and of self and identity as ever-changing and principally open and, indeed, even elusive. Against the cultural backdrop of modernity and modernism, many philosophers and artists lost the self-certainty and self-certitude characteristic of earlier times. It has often been claimed that there was a medieval self or, more generically, a Christian self that served as the counter concept to the modern self. Unlike the crisis-ridden modern subject, the Christian self appears firm and stable because it is grounded in God, and God is unchanging and eternal. That is, the fundamental condition of the Christian self dominating European Middle Ages and early modern times is that of stability, even beyond death. Thanks to the continuity of the soul there is life after death, eternal life. This is, by the way, an option for both Christian and Judeo traditions of spirituality, at least for those believers who lived a life agreeable to God. In contrast, the modern self appears to be less monolithic and more open and changeable. It is subject to the Enlightenment imperative that it has to be created (and challenged) by each individual anew: *sapere aude*—dare to know! Have the courage to use your own understanding and act accordingly. Whatever you are, it is not evident; you have to find out, you have to commit yourself; you have to create your "self," that is: your selves or "characters," as Robert Musil put the matter in the first volume of his 1930 novel *The Man Without Qualities*.

> [T]he inhabitant of a country has at least nine characters: a professional, a national, a civic, a class, a geographic, a sexual, a conscious, an unconscious, and possibly even a private character to boot. He unites them in himself, but they dissolve him, so that he is really nothing more than a small basin hollowed out by these many streamlets that trickle into it and drain out of it again, to join other such rills in filling some other basin. Which is why every inhabitant of the earth also has a tenth character that is nothing else than the passive fantasy of spaces yet unfilled. This permits a person all but one thing: to take seriously what his at least nine other characters do and what happens to them; in other words, it prevents precisely what should be his true fulfillment. (Musil, 1996, p. 30)

As Musil demonstrates by narrative means, both the concept of the self and the experienced sense of self turned more and more into a question of interpretation. The modern self—if we then still want to use this most generic and empty category—has to find out what it is. Put differently, the self fuses with the process of self-exploration, which in this context is just another word for self-interpretation. In this process, language, and especially narrative, play an important hermeneutic role—a dynamic I have pointed out elsewhere (Brockmeier, 2023).

Four

Let me turn again for a moment to the traditional view. As noted, for a long time it was common to refer to the premodern self as the original rock-solid bed that became ever more shaky the more external intruders like Copernicus, Kant, Darwin, Freud, and the like took center stage. In his study on the historical emergence of modern self-understanding, *Sources of the Self: The Origin of the Modern Identity*, Charles Taylor (1989) has rejected this assumption. He has shown that, intellectually, the erosion of the idea of a given and stable self already started much earlier, with Christianity itself. The Christian self, Taylor argues, was from the very beginning anything but stable and consistent. At all times, it was subject to doubt, conflict, and internal struggle, even if there was always the desire and hope to reach an ideal state of mind that was close to the godly sphere and free from earthly temptations and troubles. We find this feeling and yearning conjured up in sacral art and architecture. Affectively, it has been perhaps most powerfully expressed in music, such as Johann Sebastian Bach's *Passions*. Nevertheless, this great dream of a stable and balanced self is a projection of the longing for redemption and salvation; it never lost the aura of otherworldliness. When believers in a Gothic cathedral looked up they saw the vanishing points of the vaulted ceiling disappearing in an unreachable distance.

In the real world, things are messier, and so is the self. In this world, whether in medieval or modern terms, there seem to be some fundamental questions that, Taylor has argued, individuals in the West ask about themselves which cannot be sufficiently answered with any general doctrine of human nature—whether religious, philosophical, or scientific; whether referring to soul, reason, or biology. Despite all these doctrines, we still face some questions about ourselves. We roughly gesture at them using terms like "identity" and "self," as Taylor goes on to say (1989, p. 184). Yet there is no concluding scientific explanation of the meaning of my being in the world. Nor is there a philosophical system that offers a stringent theory of my existence. There remains a persisting question about me, and that is, writes Taylor, "why I think of myself as a self" (p. 184).

It is important to keep in mind that the word "self" does not refer to an existing or imagined entity. Nor does it aim at a particular quality or specific empirical form of the human being. It rather "circumscribes an area of questioning. It designates the kind of being of which this question of identity can be asked," to again use Taylor's words (p. 184).

There is another aspect of Taylor's understanding of the modern tradition of the self that is important in this context. At stake is the tradition of a self that lives and experiences its crisis as inherent to human existence. Drawing on Taylor we might say that the process of self-exploration is part and parcel of establishing one's identity. What is more, the search for one's self takes place in order to come to terms with oneself, not to tackle an external crisis or ward off an enemy intruder who challenges the health and peace of mind of an otherwise firm and stable self. There has always been an enemy to the modern self. However, this enemy is not an external threat; it is not the consequence of a virus mutation or a transfer from the animal kingdom. It is the "inner" question of meaning that emerges with the disappearance of the premodern world and the rise of capitalism and bourgeois culture.

This transformation has changed the rules of the game. The need to give meaning to one's existence has become an existential imperative. It might be augmented by putatively external crises like COVID-19; it might be triggered and brought to the fore by pandemics, but it is not generated or caused by them. Viewed in this way, my point of departure—the idea of a substantial self engaged in a struggle with an external enemy, the deadly virus—appears as a narrative scene that mingles two complex scenarios. One is the existential condition of "the Western self," the other a global pandemic out of control. This merger reduces two multi-layered cultural constellations to a simple but suggestive mythical storyline: that of a fight, man against man, or more precisely, self against virus.

Five

To finish I want to tie up some aspects of the self and its crises by discussing a film, Ingmar Bergman's *The Seventh Seal*. I saw this movie again during the long weeks and months of coronavirus lockdown. The film developed out of Bergman's play *Wood Painting* that he wrote and directed on multiple stages in the 1950s, a few years after the end of World War II. Despite its medieval setting, the film was conceived of as a modernist project—Bergman called it "an allegory of modern times"—in line with all of his earlier work. Aesthetically, *The Seventh Seal* represents the spectacular breakthrough of one of the most radical directors in film history. It tells the story of a knight, Antonius Block, who returns from a crusade to his homeland, Sweden, that is devastated by the plague. Death is everywhere. There is a historical background to this story—the pandemic that ravaged Europe in the Middle Ages killing one-third of its people.

Coming home, the knight is completely disillusioned, and his journey has turned into a search for meaning. From the beginning of the film, it is clear Death is waiting for him. The knight, however, manages to wrest his life from Death for the duration of a match of chess. He wants to use this time for "one meaningful deed" ending what he sees as a pointless and wasted life. But before he dies, he wants to know whether there is a meaning to his existence.

Well, to make it short, Block does not find the ultimate meaning of his life. He does not find an answer because even Death does not know an answer, and so Block dies unredeemed. But despite this bleak outlook and the horrors of the Black Death in the background of the plot, the knight—portrayed by the great Swedish actor Max von Sydow—is determined until the end to explore his options. Is there at least the possibility of still another layer of meaning to his life? Is there a sense, a purpose that he has not yet discovered, irrespective of the many battles he fought and lost and the many thoughts that passed his mind? Even vis-à-vis Death he keeps wondering—as if the one meaningful deed he still hopes to carry out is to keep the question open. As if he insisted that there is still a question about himself, however thorny the idea is that allows him to think about himself as a self.

Like all humans, even this mythical knight dies. But then, the film suggests, there must have been at least one moment in Block's life, an island in the flux of time, when these questions could be asked and accepted as ultimate concerns—concerns that reach further than what triggered them. In this moment, they would become, for Block, the dominant form of life itself, of being or having a self. This island surfaces during the chess match with Death. "Do you ever stop questioning?" Death asks. The knight shakes his head: "I cannot."

At the same time, Bergman's film investigates how one of the great modern myths of the self came into being: the myth of the substantial self, the sovereign subject, the Western ego that suffers from the narcissistic blows. At least for the time span of one chess match knight Antonio Block appears to be on equal footing with Death, the ultimate challenger who always wins. A few years after World War II, Italian poet Cesare Pavese wrote his poem *Verrà la morte e avrà i tuoi occhi / When death comes, it will have your eyes*, giving shape to a similar vision of death.

When death comes, it will have your eyes
This death that is always with us,
From morning till night, sleepless,
Deaf, like an old regret
Or some senseless bad habit. Your eyes
Will be a useless word,
A stifled cry, a silence.

—Cesare Pavese (1951)

One can watch Bergman's film itself as a myth-like narrative, a story about death and the different ways humans cope with it or, in this movie, with him and his principle "No one escapes me." But at the end of the day, Block rejects the myth, even though he does not have any idea of how to win the chess game of life and death. He breaks out of the romanticizing story of man fighting Death, a story quite similar to that of man fighting the virus, the patient fighting disease.

Whereas every myth is an answer to a question, Bergman leaves the question of the meaning of Block's existence unanswered, as he leaves us with the impression that the knight's life and his sense of existence cannot be distinguished from the search for his self. Thus, the film brings us to the point where we understand the dilemma of Block, and indeed of Bergmann, that the human search for meaning is endless but lifetime is not.

Note

I thank Rita Charon for our discussions on various issues of this essay.

References

Brecht, B. (1971). In the jungle of cities. In *Collected plays, Vol. 1*. Vintage.

Brockmeier, J. (2023). Verstehen and narrative. In H. Meretoja & M. Freeman (Eds.), *The use and abuse of stories: New directions in narrative hermeneutics* (pp. 89–122). Oxford University Press.

Danziger, K. (1990). *Constructing the subject: Historical origins of psychological research*. Cambridge University Press.

Freud, S. (1955). A difficulty in the path of psycho-analysis. *The Standard Edition of the Complete Psychological Works of Sigmund Freud, Volume XVII (1917–1919): An infantile neurosis and other works* (pp. 135–144). Hogarth.

Harré, R. (1998). *The singular self: An introduction to the psychology of personhood*. Sage.

Holzkamp, K. (2013). Personality: A functional analysis of the concept. In K. Holzkamp (Ed.), *Psychology from the standpoint of the subject* (pp. 77–86). Palgrave Macmillan.

James, W. (1880/1950). *The principles of psychology, Vol. 1*. Dover.

Musil, R. (1996). *The man without qualities*. Transl. by Sophie Wilkins and Burton Pike. Alfred A. Knopf (German original 1930).

Pavese, C. (1951). *Verrà la morte e avrà i tuoi occhi*. Einaudi.

Taylor, C. (1989). *Sources of the self: The making of the modern identity*. Cambridge University Press.

Index